# HORMONE-PRODUCING TUMORS
## of the GASTROINTESTINAL TRACT

# CONTEMPORARY ISSUES in GASTROENTEROLOGY VOL. 5

## SERIES EDITORS

Sidney Cohen, M.D.

Roger D. Soloway, M.D.

# HORMONE-PRODUCING TUMORS of the GASTROINTESTINAL TRACT

Edited by

## Sidney Cohen, M.D.

Chief, Gastrointestinal Section
Department of Medicine
University of Pennsylvania School of Medicine
Philadelphia, Pennsylvania

and

## Roger D. Soloway, M.D.

Associate Chief, Gastrointestinal Section
Department of Medicine
University of Pennsylvania School of Medicine
Philadelphia, Pennsylvania

**Churchill Livingstone**
**New York, Edinburgh, London, and Melbourne**
**1985**

Acquisitions editor: *Lynne Herndon*
Copy editor: *Ann Ruzycka*
Production editor: *Michiko Davis*
Production supervisor: *Kerry A. O'Rourke*
Compositor: *Kingsport Press*
Printer/Binder: *Halliday Lithograph*

Distributed in the United Kingdom by Churchill Livingstone,
Robert Stevenson House, 1–3 Baxter's Place, Leith Walk,
Edinburgh EH1 3AF and associated companies, branches
and representatives throughout the world.

First published in 1985

Printed in U.S.A.

ISBN 0-443-08370-3

9 8 7 6 5 4 3 2 1

**Library of Congress Cataloging in Publication Data**
Main entry under title:

Hormone-producing tumors of the gastrointestinal tract.

(Contemporary issues in gastroenterology; vol. 5)
Includes bibliographies and index.
1. Gastrointestinal system—Tumors.  2. Gastrointes-
tinal hormones.  I. Cohen, Sidney.
II. Soloway, Roger D.  III. Series: Contemporary issues
in gastroenterology; 5.  [DNLM: 1. Gastrointestinal
Neoplasms—secretion.  W1 CO769MQR v.5 / WI 149 H812]
RC280.D5H67  1985        616.99'233        84–17630
ISBN 0–443–08370–3

Manufactured in the United States of America

# Contributors

**Stephen R. Bloom, D.Sc., M.D., F.R.C.P.**
Professor of Endocrinology
Hammersmith Hospital
London, England

**Guenther Boden, M.D.**
Professor of Medicine
Chief, Division of Metabolism/Diabetes
Temple University School of Medicine
Philadelphia, Pennsylvania

**Francesco Carlei, M.D.**
Assistant Professor
6° Clinica Chirurgica
Policlinico Umberto 1°
Rome, Italy

**Daniel G. Haller, M.D.**
Assistant Professor of Medicine
Hematology/Oncology Section
Department of Medicine
University of Pennsylvania School of Medicine
Philadelphia, Pennsylvania

**Jens Juul Holst, M.D.**
Associate Professor
Doctor of Medical Science
Institute of Medical Physiology C
The Panum Institute
University of Copenhagen
Copenhagen, Denmark

**Bernard M. Jaffe, M.D.**
Professor and Chairman
Department of Surgery
State University of New York
Downstate Medical Center
Brooklyn, New York

**Robert T. Jensen, M.D.**
Senior Investigator
Digestive Diseases Branch
NIADDK, National Institutes of Health
Bethesda, Maryland

**Denis M. McCarthy, M.D., M.Sc., F.A.C.P.**
Professor of Medicine
University of New Mexico
Chief of Gastroenterology
Veterans Administration Medical Center
Albuquerque, New Mexico

**David McFadden, M.D.**
Assistant Clinical Instructor
Department of Surgery
State University of New York
Downstate Medical Center
Brooklyn, New York

**Hagop S. Mekhjian, M.D.**
Professor of Medicine
Department of Medicine
The Ohio State University College of Medicine
Columbus, Ohio

**Thomas M. O'Dorisio, M.D.**
Professor of Medicine
Department of Medicine
The Ohio State University College of Medicine
Columbus, Ohio

**Julia M. Polak, D.Sc., M.D., M.R.C.Path.**
Reader in Histochemistry
Hammersmith Hospital
London, England

**Ryushi Shimoyama, M.D.**
Research Fellow
Temple University School of Medicine
Philadelphia, Pennsylvania

**Aaron I. Vinik, M.D.**
Professor
Departments of Medicine and Surgery
The University of Michigan Medical School
Ann Arbor, Michigan

# Preface

Volume 5 of *Contemporary Issues in Gastroenterology* deals with the rapidly developing field of hormone-producing tumors of the gastrointestinal tract. This volume directs its attention to the major issues in understanding, diagnosing, and treating patients with these syndromes. In each chapter, acknowledged experts in this specific area of discussion provide the current state of the art, as well as their own personal feelings concerning important issues. Chapter 1 presents the basic concepts of regulatory peptides of the gastrointestinal tract and the neoplastic origin of endocrine tumors. The chapters on gastrinoma, somatostatinoma, VIPoma, and glucagonoma provide the classical presentation of these illnesses and deal with the complexities of treatment. The chapter on Zollinger–Ellison syndrome, the most common hormone-producing tumor syndrome, provides a rational approach to the many complexities of medical and surgical treatment that have been proposed in recent years. Special attention is given to the mixed-polypeptide-producing tumors, a more recently recognized phenomenon.

The final two chapters deal with current aspects of chemotherapeutic or surgical treatment of hormone-producing tumors.

The rapid development of identifiable, biologically active peptide hormones and neurotransmitters within the gastrointestinal tract would imply that additional syndromes related to these hormones will be described in future years. The hormone-producing tumors of the gastrointestinal tract are relatively rare causes of disease in man. However, these conditions have provided greater understanding of the actions of peptides in the gastrointestinal tract and the pathogenesis of disease in man. Further understanding of these neoplastic disorders may provide insight into other gastrointestinal disorders related to hormone release or action.

*Sidney Cohen, M.D.*

# Contents

# HORMONE-PRODUCING TUMORS
# of the GASTROINTESTINAL TRACT

# 1 | Regulatory Peptides of the Gastrointestinal Tract and Their Derivative Tumors

*Francesco Carlei*
*Stephen R. Bloom*
*Julia M. Polak*

## INTRODUCTION

The possibility that digestive functions were subject to endocrine regulation was clearly demonstrated at the beginning of this century by the discovery of secretin[1] and gastrin.[2] Furthermore, many other substances, mostly peptides, able to regulate the physiological activities of gut and pancreas, have been identified and, somewhat surprisingly, these peptides and amines have subsequently been detected both in endocrine cells and nerves through the entire body.

According to their peculiar anatomical distribution these substances have been shown to act as circulating hormones (endocrine) but also as local regulators (paracrine) or neurotransmitters or all of these. For these reasons the term regulatory peptides[3] has recently been suggested to describe them.

The presence of regulatory peptides has been clearly demonstrated in the gut, where they are localized in endocrine cells scattered throughout the mucosa and in ganglion cell bodies and nerves within the gut wall.

Endocrine cells and nerves of the gut and other types of parenchyma were combined under the umbrella of the "diffuse neuroendocrine system" as a major regulatory system affecting almost all the physiological activities of the body and particularly the digestive functions.[4] The importance of this system in the understanding of many pathological conditions has come to light.

## ENDOCRINE CELLS OF THE GUT AND PANCREAS

The endocrine activity of typical clear cells scattered through different organs, particularly the gut, was first postulated by Feyrter in 1938.[5] The occurrence of electron-dense secretory granules in these cells further supported their endocrine nature,[6] while Pearse, in 1968,[7] observing their common biochemical and histochemical features, proposed the acronym APUD (*A*mine or *A*mine *P*recursor *U*ptake and/or *D*ecarboxylation) for this system of cells.

Up to twenty years ago, gut endocrine cells were visualized only by specialized histological stains such as silver impregnation,[8] lead hematoxylin,[9] aldehyde fuchsin for B cells of the pancreas, formaldehyde-induced fluorescence, and the argentaffin or diazonium methods for 5-HT-containing cells.[10]

### Electron Microscopy

More recently, the endocrine nature and the specific ultrastructural features of different endocrine cell types have been established,[11] mostly by conventional electron microscopy. Using these techniques, gut endocrine cells have been found

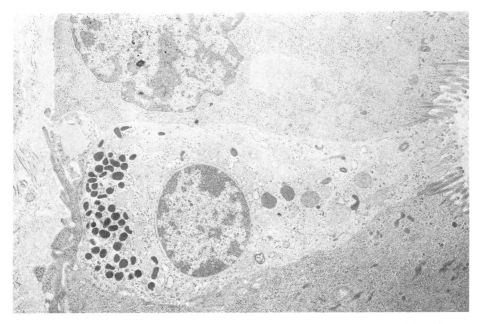

**Fig. 1-1.**   Conventional electron micrograph of an "open-type" endocrine cell from human duodenal mucosa. Glutaraldehyde-fixed, counterstained with uranyl acetate and lead citrate. (×8,190)

from the cardia to the anus widely scattered in the mucosal layer; they are usually pyramidal in form and can be roughly divided into "open" or "closed" types, since some of them exhibit a cytoplasmic process reaching the digestive lumen while others do not.[12] Ultrastructural studies show that the basal cytoplasm of these cells contains secretory granules. The synthesis of these granules appears to start in the Golgi apparatus whence they travel toward the basal portion of the cell while increasing in size. The secretory granules are extruded from the cells by exocytosis[12] (Figs. 1-1, 1-2); thus their content is released in "quanta," which is important since different substances with different activities are likely to be stored in the same granule.[13] Neurocrine, paracrine, and/or endocrine effects may therefore be related to the secretory activity of a single kind of endocrine cell. Different kinds of endocrine cell have been recognized on the basis of the typical ultrastructural characteristics of their secretory granules (e.g., size, electron-density, peripheral halo (Fig. 1-3).[11]

Different types of secretory granule can sometimes be found in a single endocrine cell of the gut.[14] It is important to point out that the number of secretory granules observed in a cell is the result of several different specific metabolic processes: (1) synthesis of the bioactive peptide, usually in the form of a larger, precursor molecule; (2) its packaging and storage in the granules together with other substances such as biogenic monoamines, ATP and/or other adenine nucleotides, metallic ions ($Ca^{++}$) and a compound protein; and (3) secretory activity of the

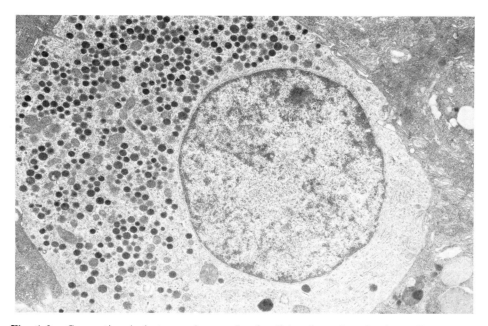

**Fig. 1-2.** Conventional electron micrograph of a "closed-type" endocrine cell, possibly $D_1$, from human ileal mucosa. Glutaraldehyde-fixed, counterstained with uranyl acetate and lead citrate. ($\times$8,190)

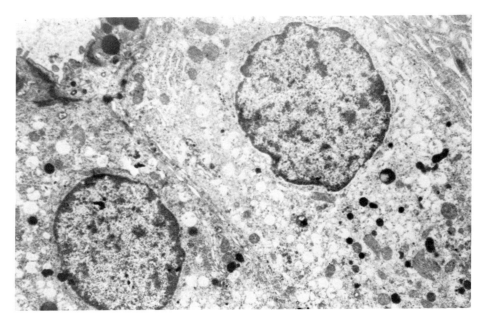

**Fig. 1-3.** Electron micrograph of adjacent gastrin-containing (G) cells from gastric mucosa of man. Cells contain two distinct types of secreting granules, small (160nm) electron-dense and large (240nm) electron-lucent. Glutaraldehyde-fixed, counterstained with uranyl acetate and lead citrate. (×6,550)

cell by exocytosis in response to different stimuli. It is believed that in endocrine cells having a high rate of secretory activity the granule content will be extremely scanty, while it will be increased in resting metabolic conditions.

Ultrastructural studies have demonstrated microvilli on the luminal border of endocrine cells of open type[12] (Fig. 1-1). It is believed that chemical receptors are located in the tuft of microvilli, regulating the metabolic activity of the cell in response to chemical and environmental stimuli from the lumen.[15,16]

In addition to responding to external forces, endocrine cells of the gut are also governed by inter-regulatory mechanisms as shown by the finding of morphological and functional connections between different types of endocrine cells or endocrine cells and nerves in the gut and pancreas.[9,17,18,19,20]

## Immunocytochemistry

The advent of immunocytochemical techniques truly revolutionized the recognition and the characterization of the endocrine component of the gut. Using a wide range of antibodies raised against different peptides or specific portions of their molecules, it has at last been possible to demonstrate these substances within the endocrine cells (Fig. 1-4) and, by the use of semithin-thin-sectioning techniques, to correlate their presence with the electron microscopical features of the cells

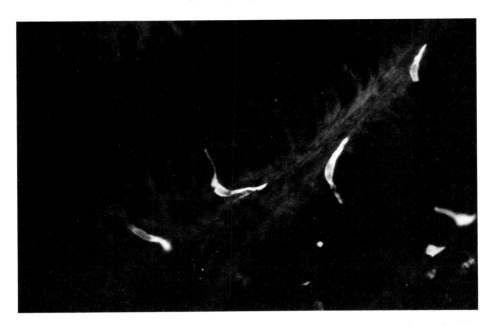

**Fig. 1-4.** Enteroglucagon-immunoreactive cells in human ileum. Benzoquinone fixation, indirect immunofluorescence method. (×365)

(Fig. 1-5). Finally, new techniques for immunocytochemistry at the electron micro-scope level such as the immunogold procedure[21] that can reveal several antigens simultaneously have made possible the identification of the metabolic pathways leading to hormone synthesis, processing, and secretion.[22,23,24]

However, since different peptides can share one or more amino acid sequences, one must consider the possibility of cross reactions when dealing with immunochem-ical methods. Other causes of error or pitfalls in immunocytochemistry are related to inadequate antigen fixation and non-specific binding to the tissue of antiserum components; finally, one must always take care when dealing with the recognition of larger precursor molecules of the final peptide, since the immunoreactive sites may be considerably modified during intracellular processing.

## Neuron-Specific Enolase (NSE) for the Demonstration of the Diffuse Neuroendocrine System

There are still several histochemically and ultrastructurally characterized en-docrine cell types producing and storing unknown or uncharacterized substances.[11] It is evident that these products cannot yet be revealed by immunochemical tech-niques. It is thus particularly important that all neuroendocrine structures (cells and nerves) of the body, including the endocrine cells of the gut, exhibit a common marker, namely the enzyme responsible for energy provision through the glycolytic pathways, neuron-specific enolase (NSE). This enzyme, originally thought to be

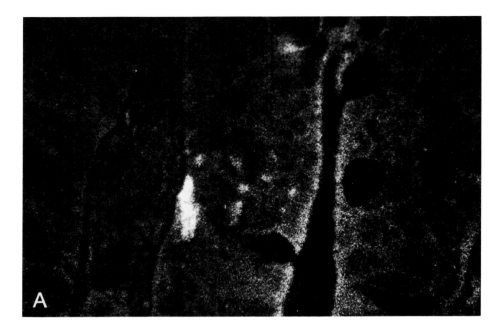

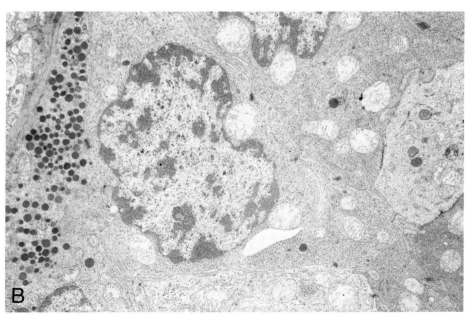

**Fig. 1-5.** (A) Somatostatin immunoreactive endocrine cell in human colnic mucosa. Glutar-aldehyde-fixed, $2\mu$ resin section. Indirect immunofluorescence method. ($\times2,340$) (B) Corresponding ultrathin section of (A). ($\times8,190$)

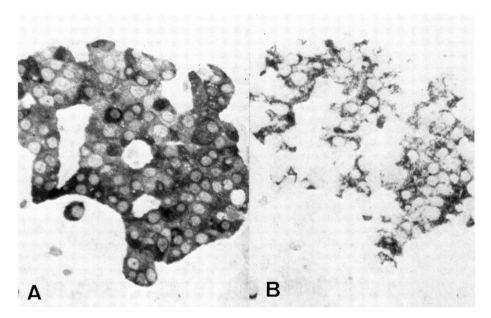

**Fig. 1-6.** Human pancreatic islet immunostained for (A) neuron specific enolase (NSE) and (B) insulin. Benzoquinone fixation, peroxidase/antiperoxidase method. ($\times$365)

confined to neurons, is the most acidic of the enolase isoenzymes, all of which are dimers, containing 2 of the 3 known subunits ($\alpha$, $\beta$ and $\gamma$).[24a] NSE consists of 2 $\gamma\gamma$ subunits of 39 K° each. NSE, detected first in nerves of the central nervous system, appears to be present in all neuroendocrine components, cells, and nerves, but not in other tissues. Thus the demonstration of NSE by immuno-chemical methods is the simplest and most reliable way of delineating neuroendo-crine structures in health and disease (Fig. 1-6).[24b] Other neuronal and non-neuronal brain-specific proteins may also be markers for the endocrine component of the gut.

Another highly acidic brain protein, named S-100 and first described in astro-cytes and glial cells,[25] has been found in myelinated nerves and glial cells of the diffuse neuroendocrine system of the gut.[26] It is conceivable that there will be changes in S-100 content in degenerative or regenerative processes affecting the innervation of the gut.

## HYPERPLASIA OF GUT ENDOCRINE CELLS

Hyperplastic changes of different endocrine cell types have frequently been mentioned by many authors. One of the most important problems concerns the quantification of the changes, since the analysis made by the observer is subjective. Various morphometric methods have been suggested, taking into account several parameters such as tissue orientation, section thickness, and distribution of endocrine cells at different levels, all of which have to be checked in order to avoid false interpretation of the results.[27] Computerized image analyzing systems are now available to aid quantification and statistical analysis.

Endocrine hyperplasias of the gut can be described as diffuse, focal, regularly or irregularly distributed through the mucosa, intraepithelial or endophytic (protruding into the lamina propria), and related to orthotopic or metaplastic epithelia.

Enterochromaffin-like (ECL) cell hyperplasia has been postulated in patients with non-neoplastic pathological conditions such as hyperchlorhydria and duodenal ulcer with moderate hypergastrinemia. In patients with Zollinger-Ellison syndrome, ECL cell hyperplasia of the oxyntic portion of the stomach is prominent.[28,29,30] Gastrin-cell hyperplasia can sometimes be observed in duodenal ulcer disease with food-stimulated hypergastrinemia, while it is more often present in achlorhydric patients with pernicious anemia and fundic gastritis.[31,32]

A trophic action of the substance produced by the apudoma cannot be excluded, as in the case of parietal cell hyperplasia[33] with typical hyperplastic gastritis[34] in patients with gastrinoma.

Hyperplasia of ECL cells is also present in these cases. Although micronodular and extraepithelial spread of endocrine cells can sometimes be observed, the oncological potential of these conditions is considered to be slight.

Nevertheless, the occurrence of gastrin-secreting tumors in 2 patients[35,36] with antral G cell hyperplasia and also the multifocal nature of gastrinomas[37] suggests that these tumors may develop from G cell hyperplasias. The presence of hyperplastic growths is not always demonstrable, since cases of severe antral G cell hyperfunction with barely augmented G cell mass have been described.[38] Although gastritis-associated endocrine hyperplasia can be considered benign, multiple argyrophilic carcinoids have been detected in patients affected by chronic atrophic gastritis, as have all intermediate conditions from nodular hyperplasia to neoplasia.[39] Hyperplasia of small intestinal endocrine cells has been very seldom described; one example is provided by cases of coeliac disease,[40] while ECL micronodular hyperplasia has been described in patients with "neuroendocrine" appendicitis.[40a]

## GUT ENDOCRINE TUMORS: APUDOMAS

### General Characteristics of Apudomas

The term apudoma covers all neoplasias that are derived from APUD cells and have all the associated biochemical and histochemical features described by Pearse.[7]

The importance of the APUD theory in understanding the many different aspects of gut endocrine tumors justifies the use of this term, even when it is used to describe neoplasias of extremely different patterns. Even so, the advantages of this classification outweigh the disadvantages. For instance, the assessment of certain common features (biochemical, histological, clinical, etc.) required by the apudoma concept has suddenly given light to uninterpreted cases that had not been convincingly explained by the classical theories of gastroenterology.

It must be recognized that the term "apudoma" does not imply any strict morphological or histopathological criteria and that the terms by which most apudomas are described (insulinoma, gastrinoma, glucagonoma, somatostatinoma, etc.) were based upon the name of the peptide originally thought to be responsible for the associated syndrome.

We can roughly distinguish two different groups of apudoma patients. The first "sporadic" group consists of young or middle aged (below 50) people, apparently previously in good health. A family history of endocrine disorders is not uncommon, so that retrospective analysis and careful follow-up of relatives is obviously mandatory. The second group of apudoma patients is composed of younger people with inherited endocrine disease caused by an autosomal dominant gene with a high degree of penetrance. The disease consists of multiple endocrine tumors variably affecting different glands.[41,42]

This second group of patients must be considered separately from the first, since it involves different etiological concepts and different diagnostic and therapeutic approaches. Although apudomas are usually associated with a clinical syndrome, there are some apudomas of the gut lacking any paraneoplastic symptoms, for example, most of the malignant carcinoids of the hindgut.[43]

The apudomas not associated with clinical syndromes may be highly malignant tumors associated with extremely poor prognosis. In these cases it is likely that the neoplastic cells are not able to produce and release any bioactive substance. Alternatively, they could synthesize an abnormal product with considerably altered structure in the bioactive part of the molecule. A third possibility is that the tumor could produce two or more substances with mutually antagonistic effects.

## Multiple-Hormone-Producing Tumors

A polysecreting tumor was first recognized in 1959 when an endocrine tumor of the pancreas secreting both ACTH and insulin was reported,[44] but since then it has been accepted that apudomas usually produce more than one peptide.[45] One peptide in particular occurs quite commonly in apudomas and its presence in abnormal amounts in the blood stream has been considered as a possible marker for the screening of apudomas. This peptide, pancreatic polypeptide (PP), was detected in a significantly higher percentage than other known regulatory peptides in a series of pancreatic tumors, while its circulating levels in blood were significantly elevated.[46] It appears that different populations of neoplastic endocrine cells are usually present in apudomas. This has been convincingly proved by light microscopical immunocytochemistry and also by electron microscopical observation (Fig. 1-7).[47] Similarly, radioimmunoassay analysis of tissue extracts often confirms the presence of different bioactive substances in the neoplastic tissue. It also appears relatively common that different regulatory peptides are produced, stored, and released by the same neoplastic cell. Immunochemical techniques have been conclusive in such cases, although even by conventional electron microscopy it is often possible to visualize an extremely large variety of different secretory granules in the cytoplasm of apudoma cells.[48] It is well known that the most striking clinical feature in apudoma patients is the presence of a typical syndrome sustained by

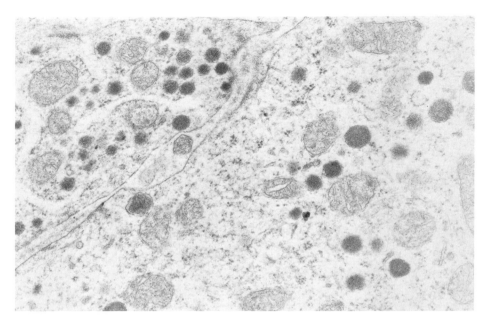

**Fig. 1-7.** VIP-producing tumor from jejunum of man. Two distinct populations of secretory granules are present in adjacent cells. Glutaraldehyde-fixed, counterstained with uranyl acetate and lead citrate. (×30,130)

pathologically high levels of a specific bioactive substance produced by the neoplastic cells. Other chapters of this book are devoted to the description of most apudoma syndromes.

However, this kind of general scheme does not fully explain the complex biochemical and clinical pattern of apudomas.

In fact, in many instances, plasma and tissue levels of the peptide produced by the tumor cannot be related to the severity of the symptoms or cannot explain one of the symptoms constantly associated with the syndrome. For example, in glucagonoma patients, glucagon levels do not correlate with the severity of the impairment of glucose metabolism and, moreover, they do not explain the typical skin lesions constantly present in these patients.[49,50] There are several reasons for these discrepancies: the apudomas may be producing substances not yet identified and therefore not measurable in the plasma or the tissue, or the substance produced by the tumor is not identical in its chemical composition and biological activity to the normal counterpart produced by euplastic endocrine cells. In fact, neoplastic endocrine cells in apudomas often secrete larger molecules similar to the precursors that are usually detected only at intracellular levels in normal conditions.[51,52] This may be because the neoplastic cells lack a proper mechanism for packaging and storing these substances,[48] or the metabolic cleavage from larger molecular precursors that usually takes place in the secretory granules may be absent in neoplastic endocrine cells.

It has been reported that after a certain period apudomas are able to change their type of secretion and that different secretory activity can take place in the primary tumor compared to its metastasis.[45,53] The explanation for these almost unknown aspects of the pathophysiology of apudomas may be the key to understanding their cellular behavior and improving the therapeutic approach.

## Frequency

The availability of advanced techniques such as immunohistochemistry and radioimmunoassay and their use in the clinical management of patients affected by common gastrointestinal and pancreatic disturbances such as peptic ulcer or diabetes have shown that apudomas are by no means exceptional occurrences.

Until recently, their discovery was hampered by inadequate laboratory techniques or inappropriate diagnostic tests. Nevertheless, there appears to be a wide discrepancy in the occurrence of different kinds of apudoma syndrome. The occurrence of carcinoids, insulinomas, and gastrinomas is much more frequent than that of the few cases of other apudoma syndromes reported (somatostatinomas,[54] neurotensinomas, etc.).

The best example is Zollinger-Ellison syndrome, now known to be due to a gastrinoma. Since its discovery in 1955[54a] and the parallel improvement of immunochemical techniques, the number of cases detected every year has risen consistently. However, we must still take into account the poor definition of the clinical picture and the difficulties in assessment of the biochemical parameters required for the diagnosis of many apudoma syndromes.

## DIAGNOSTIC CRITERIA

## Evaluation of Biochemical Parameters

Another extremely difficult task is the interpretation of laboratory tests performed to assess the existence of an apudoma. Elevated plasma levels of a particular peptide can be due to causes other than an endocrine tumor. An immediate example is the hypergastrinemia almost always present in patients with pernicious anemia and chronic atrophic gastritis,[55] but other conditions such as retained or excluded antral tissue after gastrectomy[56] are also associated with recurrent peptic ulcer and elevated plasma gastrin levels. The differential diagnosis of gastrinomas is certainly a hard task for the clinician.

An important feature of neoplastic endocrine cells is their ability to exhibit secretory activity after administration of specific substances, for example metallic ions such as calcium, amino acids, other polypeptides, secretin, and gastrin.[57] These substances may act in a different manner on non-neoplastic endocrine cells. These tests, too, require careful interpretation.

## Pathology of Apudomas

Until twenty years ago the assessment of the endocrine nature of a tumor of the gastrointestinal tract and the pancreas was made mainly upon its histopathological features. In most instances these tumors are formed by round, polygonal, or occasionally spindle-shaped neoplastic cells with clear cytoplasm typically containing fine secretory granules. These granules are stainable by various histochemical methods. The mitotic activity and nuclear pleomorphism is usually slight, as is the degree of infiltration into the surrounding non-neoplastic tissue, the blood vessels, and the lymphatic spaces. A capsule of fibrotic tissue often surrounds the tumor. The size of the tumor may also be prognostic. For instance, carcinoids more than two centimeters in diameter are always considered malignant.[57] The neoplastic cells are distributed in various spatial arrangements described as rosette-like, nests, ribbons, or branching (Fig. 1-8). The histological features may vary in different regions of the same apudoma. Coarse strands of connective tissue containing blood vessels divide the neoplastic cells; the amount of fibrosis is extremely variable. Necrotic and hemorrhagic areas are very rarely observed.

Although the above listed pathological aspects are often seen in gut apudomas, great variability is also the rule. Tumors with mixed populations of neoplastic cells, scanty or extremely poorly granulated cytoplasm, and highly malignant behavior previously recorded as undifferentiated carcinomas or lymphomas have now been classified as apudomas.

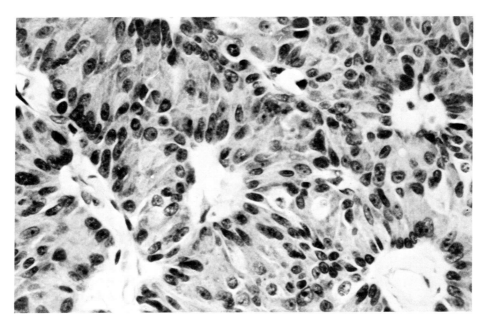

**Fig. 1-8.** Hematoxylin-eosin staining of a pancreatic apudoma, showing the typical ribbon-like arrangement of the cells. Formalin fixation. (×410)

## Electron Microscopy

The use of conventional electron microscopy provided a major step forward in the histological assessment of apudomas, since cytoplasmic secretory granules could be identified even when they were so scanty as to be undetectable using light microscopy. Moreover, by analyzing specific parameters (shape, size, halo) of the granules, it is sometimes possible to correlate the different types of secretory granule of the neoplastic cells with different peptides.

## Histochemical Methods

Many endocrine neoplasms can be recognized by use of appropriate techniques such as argyrophilic staining (Grimelius method)[8] (Fig. 1-9) and lead-hematoxylin.[58] Aldehyde-fuchsin may be useful in the diagnosis of pancreatic B cell tumors.

Formaldehyde-induced-fluorescence[10] and the argentaffin and diazonium reactions have been used for 5-HT-containing tumors. However, the possibility of recognizing the endocrine nature of neoplastic growths using these techniques is often related to the number of granules stored in the cytoplasm. Since neoplastic cells often lack a proper mechanism for storing their products, the classical staining methods may be ineffective. Moreover, most of the staining methods do not give any information about the chemical nature of the peptide produced by the neoplasm.

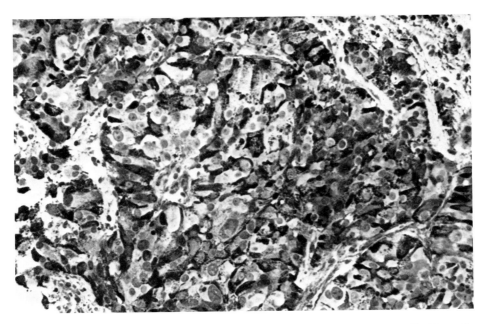

**Fig. 1-9.** Pancreatic apudoma showing positive silver staining in numerous cells. Formalin fixation, argyrophilic silver impregnation method. (×365)

### Immunocytochemistry

However, the ultimate step in the histochemical assessment of apudomas has been immunocytochemistry. Using a large number of region-specific antibodies for all known peptides and other tumor products, we are now able to recognize peptides, amines, and enzymes in apudoma cells. In the past few years immunocytochemistry has also been applied at the electron microscopical level, especially with the use of gold labelling techniques.[21] With these methods we are now able to identify the intracellular localization of most peptides and their precursors (Fig. 1-10).

Another problem of crucial importance is the difference between what we are able to detect and to measure by immunochemical methods and the real bioactivity of a substance in vivo, since these techniques detect any substance with similar immunoreactivity to the natural or synthetic substance against which the antibody was raised. The use of newly discovered techniques and progress in immunochemical methods will create a major improvement in this respect. Monoclonal antibodies, in particular, will be extremely useful in the detection of poorly characterized substances.[59]

Even when a peptide cannot be positively identified, the use of antibodies to the enzyme marker, NSE, will allow a tumor to be classified as a neuroendocrine neoplasm[60] (Fig. 1-11), or as an area of neuroendocrine hyperplasia to be defined.

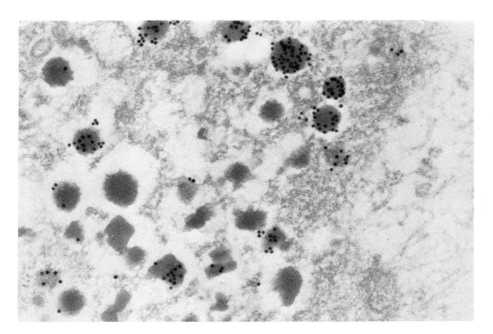

**Fig. 1-10.** C-peptide immunoreactive secretory granules in insulin-containing cell from insulinoma. A sub-population of granules are immunoreactive (arrowed). Glutaraldehyde-fixed, counterstained with uranyl acetate and lead citrate. (×51,300)

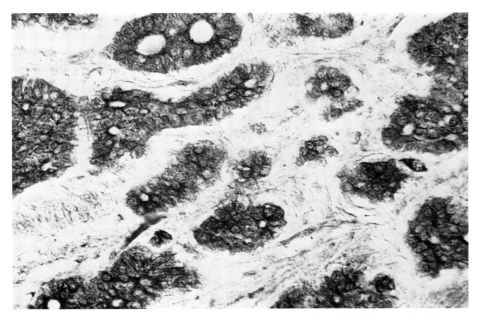

**Fig. 1-11.** Strong immunoreactivity for neuron specific enolase (NSE) in a carcinoid tumor. Benzoquinone fixation, peroxidase/antiperoxidase method. (×286)

Moreover, NSE immunodetection can be carried out on conventionally fixed and paraffin-embedded material, allowing the possibility of retrospective studies. The intracellular presence of NSE is not related to the granule content, so that NSE detection is possible even in poorly granulated endocrine tumors.

## INDIVIDUAL CLINICAL SYNDROMES

### Gastrinomas

About 1% of gastrinomas arise from the stomach, upper jejunum, and biliary tree, 13% from the duodenum, and 85% from the pancreas.[61] These observations do not fit with the physiological occurrence of G cells in the digestive system[39]; however, during development G cells appear first in the duodenum and they are also present in the pancreas of fetal rats.[62] Malignancy occurs more often in pancreatic gastrinomas (62% or even more) than in duodenal gastrinomas (38%).[63] Two main types of G cell have been identified on the basis of their ultrastructural features and their immunoreactivity[39]: the pyloric type (G) shows vesicular granules reacting with antigastrin G17, while the intestinal type (IG) has smaller, solid granules resembling the Golgi-associated progranules of pyloric G cells. Both these types are commonly present in gastrinomas (Fig. 1-12).[24]

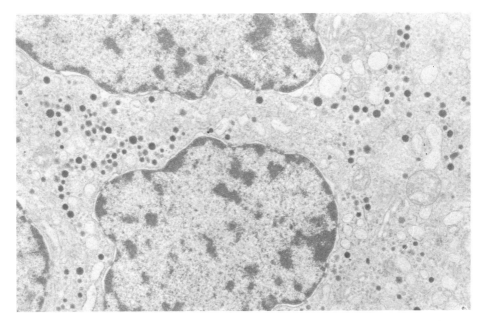

**Fig. 1-12.**   Gastrin-producing tumor (gastrinoma) from pancreas of man. A range of secretory granule types are present in the cells though they are predominantly of the intestinal gastrin type. Glutaraldehyde-fixed, counterstained with uranyl acetate and lead citrate. (×12,800)

In some tumors large, dense, and irregular granules may be detected together with G or IG type granules[64]; such granules might contain the corticotrophin-like peptides that have been described, mainly by one worker, in euplastic antral G cells.[64a]

## Insulinomas

Beta cell tumors are the most common endocrine tumors of the pancreas; even with small adenomas hypoglycemic disturbances are almost invariably present, but fortunately more than 85% of them are benign.[65] Although they are very often well differentiated, their cells may contain fewer granules than normal β-cells, smaller and sometimes atypical, and they often contain more proinsulin.[66]

## Glucagonomas

Although non-argentaffin carcinoids of the large bowel containing L-type cells resembling the enteroglucagon-producing L cells of the normal large bowel often react with non-C terminal antiglucagon antibodies,[67] the term glucagonoma is restricted to endocrine tumors localized almost always in the pancreas (Fig. 1-13). In most cases they are malignant, containing pancreatic glucagon and associated

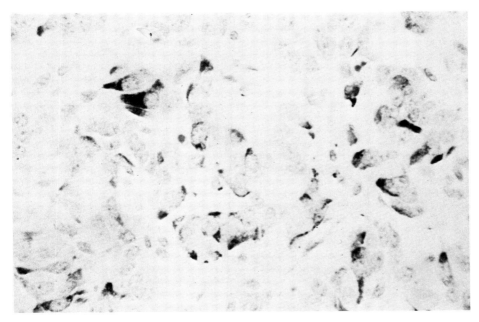

**Fig. 1-13.** Numerous glucagon-immunoreactive cells in a glucagonoma. Benzoquinone fixation, peroxidase/anti-peroxidase method. (×410)

with a typical syndrome (diarrhea, anemia, hyperglycemia, glossitis and skin rash).[49] In these tumors target-like A granules as well as non diagnostic homogeneous type of granule are very often present.[68] Small, clinically silent A-cell adenomas can be found incidentally during autopsy.[69]

## Diarrheogenic Tumors

Although most endocrine tumors are associated with diarrhea,[70] the term diarrheogenic tumor has been more often used to describe the syndrome associated with vasoactive intestinal polypeptide (VIP)-producing tumors[6]; although some of them, such as ganglioneuroblastomas, are found outside the digestive tract,[71] the so-called "VIPomas" of the gut, usually localized in the pancreas, never show a neuronal component but sometimes have an atypical carcinoid-like appearance. They are usually poorly differentiated and malignant. VIP-immunoreactivity is present in these cases; moreover, "VIPomas" also contain *p*eptide *h*istidine *i*soleucine (PHI) immunoreactivity.[71a]

PHI is a newly discovered peptide[72] having striking molecular and also biological similarities to VIP; for these reasons it has been postulated that PHI may also be involved in the causality of the *w*atery *d*iarrhea *h*ypokalemia *a*clorhydria (WDHA) syndrome. Recently, the colocalization of VIP and PHI in the same apudomas has been explained by the finding that both these peptides are coded by a single coding gene.[73,74] Approximately 10% of VIPomas and a smaller percentage of other types of pancreatic tumor are also found to secrete neurotensin.[75,76] There is no clinical consequence yet discovered of permanently elevated circulating neurotensin concentrations. Column chromatography demonstrates the molecular form to be closely similar to that normally secreted from the ileum and so presumably biologically active.

Small, round D1 type granules or larger, irregular granules are detected in "VIPomas."[13] It is of interest that additional, osmiophilic, bodies resembling Weiber-Palade bodies of the endothelium, have been described in diarrheogenic tumors; these structures might contain prostaglandin-like substances, since it has been suggested that prostaglandins play a role in endocrine cases of diarrhea.[61]

## Somatostatin (D Cell) Tumors

Somatostatin (D cell) tumors associated with a particular syndrome (diabetes, biliary stones, etc.) are extremely rare,[54] although D cells are very often present in different endocrine tumors.

## Pancreatic Tumors Producing Growth Hormone-Releasing Factor (GRF) Associated with Acromegaly

Since the recognition of Frohman and co-workers[77] in 1980 of the existence of pancreatic tumors producing extra pituitary GRF associated with acromegaly, there has been an intense search for a so-called growth hormone-releasing factor. In 1982 two separate groups[78,79] were able to chemically characterize a regulatory peptide of 40[79] or 44[78] amino acids displaying growth hormone-releasing properties. Analysis of its amino acid sequence revealed sequence homologies with peptides of the so-called glucagon-secretin family, in particular the latest member, PHI.[72] Since then there have been many reports of pancreatic endocrine tumors producing clinical features of acromegaly and characterized by the production and release of growth hormone-releasing factor. These tumors are histologically classified as classical apudomas.

## Carcinoids

These tumors are considered to derive from the Kulchitsky cell of the small intestine and are typically argentaffin[79a]; although endocrine tumors arising from sites other than the small intestine have been reported with clinical and biochemical features of the carcinoid syndrome (flushing, diarrhea, bronchoconstriction, heart failure), they are usually non-argentaffin, being argyrophilic in the foregut and non-reactive to silver stains in the hindgut. Electron microscopy shows pleomorphic, uniformly dense secretory granules.[57] Carcinoids are usually slow growing, but they tend to metastasize, producing the typical symptoms.

# CONCLUSIONS

The impressive progress achieved in the past decade in understanding endocrine mechanisms regulating gastrointestinal and pancreatic physiology have certainly made possible the identification of an increasing number of endocrine tumors of the gut. Improvements have also been achieved in the therapeutic management of apudoma patients.

As in the treatment of other neoplastic diseases, surgery is considered the ultimate therapy. Nevertheless, spectacular progress has been made in the medical field. New chemotherapeutic agents such as streptozotocin or 5 fluoro-uracil (5FU) have been successfully used in antiblastic therapy; unfortunately specific antagonists able to neutralize the systemic effects of regulatory peptides are not yet available, but various other substances have been used, particularly in the management of the symptoms such as diarrhea, hyperchlorhydria, and cardiovascular disorders. Among these substances, $H_2$ blockers are the best medical procedure for patients with gastric hyperacidity due to a gastrinoma. Moreover, somatostatin,[80] a hypothalamic and gut polypeptide possessing wide inhibitory activity on different target organs, including most endocrine cell types, has been shown also to inhibit the systemic effects produced by the apudomas.[80a,81] Somatostatin may act in different manners; lowering the releasing activity of the neoplastic cells and/or antagonizing the peripheral effects of the neoplastic mediator on the target organs. The assessment of the effects of somatostatin and other substances such as "growth factors" on the mitotic and metabolic activity of endocrine cells and their neoplastic lines may lead to revolutionary changes in the therapeutic management of apudomas.

The improvement scored in molecular biology and genetic engineering has now given us the possibility of isolating and identifying the genetic code responsible for the synthesis of different peptides and their precursors. The whole precursor molecule and the various sequences subsequently cleaved at intracellular level can now be fully characterized.[82] The more extensive use of these techniques in gut endocrinology will certainly lead to new achievements in understanding not only the metabolic pathways of peptide synthesis but also the phylogenetic evolution of peptides and the pathological changes that occur at intracellular level in neoplastic and non-neoplastic endocrine disorders.

The isolation of messenger RNA from neoplastic cells and the synthesis of complementary DNA, able to reproduce the specific peptide if inserted into a plasmid-bacteria system[82] will allow extremely specific assessment of the molecular composition of apudoma products.

Finally, the proper sequencing and cloning of the DNA strain synthesizing any peptide will facilitate the production of large amounts of the substance, solving the problems connected with denaturation of the material during extraction procedures and allowing for the possibility of therapeutic use.

Other important goals to be achieved may be listed as follows: the complete identification of endocrine cell products in neoplastic and non-neoplastic conditions, the assessment of their biological effects, and the synthesis of specific agonists and antagonists.

Clinical and pathological characterization of a larger numer of endocrine neoplasias will elucidate some of the unsolved problems concerning the cellular origin, pathology, and pathophysiology of the apudomas of the gut.

## REFERENCES

1. Bayliss WM, Starling EH: The mechanism of pancreatic secretion. J Physiol 28:325–353, 1902
2. Edkins JS: On the chemical mechanism of gastric secretion. Proc Roy Soc (London) 76:376, 1906
3. Polak JM, Bloom SR: Regulatory peptides: Key factors in the control of body function. Brit Med J 286:1461–1466, 1983
4. Polak JM, Bloom SR: The diffuse neuroendocrine system. J Histochem Cytochem 27:1398–1400, 1979
5. Feyrter F: Uber Diffuse Endokrine Epitheliale Organe. Leipzig, JA Barth, pp. 6–16, 1938
6. Bloom SR, Polak JM, Pearse AGE: Vasoactive intestinal polypeptide and watery-diarrhea syndrome. Lancet 2:14, 1973
7. Pearse AGE: Common cytochemical and ultrastructural characteristics of cells producing polypeptide hormones (the APUD series) and their relevance to thyroid and ultimobranchial C-cells and calcitonin. Proc Roy Soc (London) 170:71, 1968
8. Grimelius L: A silver nitrate stain for $a_2$ cells in human pancreatic islets. Acta Soc Med Upsallen 73:243, 1968
9. Bloom SR, Polak JM: Control of pancreatic hormone release by islet innervation. In: Current Views on Hypoglicaemia and Glucagon. Adreani D, Lefebvre PJ, Marks V, eds. London, Academic Press, 1980, p. 37–46.
10. Solcia E, Sampietro R, Capella C: Differential staining of catecholamines, 5-hydroxytryptamine and related compounds in aldehyde-fixed tissues. Histochemie 17:273, 1969
11. Solcia E, Polak JM, Larsson LI, et al.: Update on Lausanne classification of endocrine cells. In: Gut Hormones, 2nd Edition, SR Bloom and JM Polak, eds. Edinburgh, Churchill Livingstone, 1981, p. 96–100.
12. Fujita T, Kobayashi S: The endocrine cell. In: Gut Hormones, 2nd Edition, Bloom SR and Polak JM, eds. Edinburgh, Churchill Livingstone, 1981
13. Capella C, Solcia E, Frigerio B et al.: The endocrine cells of the pancreas and related tumours. Virchows Arch A. 373:327, 1977
14. Jaffe BM: Prostaglandins and serotonin in diarrheogenic syndromes. In: Gastrointestinal hormones and pathology of the digestive system. Grossman M, Speranza V, Basso N, Lezoche E, eds. New York, Plenum Press, 1978, p. 285
15. Fujita T, Kobayashi S: The cells and hormones of the GEP endocrine system—The current of studies. In: Gastro-entero-pancreatic endocrine system. A cell-biological approach. Fujita T, ed. Tokyo, Igaku Shoin, 1973, p. 1–16
16. Fujita T, Kobayashi S: Structure and function of gut endocrine cells. Int Rev Cytol (suppl) 6:187–233, 1977
17. Adrian TE, Bloom SR, Hermansen, K, et al.: Pancreatic polypeptide, glucagon and insulin secretion from the isolated perfused canine pancreas. Diabetologia 14:413–417, 1978

18. Bloom SR, Edwards AV: Pancreatic endocrine responses to stimulation of the peripheral ends of the splanchnic nerves in the conscious adrenalectomized calf. J Physiol 308:39–48, 1980

19. Eklund S, Fahrenkrug J, Jodal M, et al.: Vasoactive intestinal polypeptide, 5-hydroxy-tryptamine and reflex hyperaemia in the small intestine of the rat. J Physiol 302:549–557, 1980

20. Walsh JH: Gastrin. In: Gut Hormones, 2nd edition. SR Bloom and JM Polak, eds. Edinburgh, Churchill Livingstone, 1981

21. Varndell IM, Tapia FJ, Probert L, et al.: Immunogold staining procedure for the localization of regulatory peptides. Peptides 3:259–272, 1982

22. Ravazzola M, Orci L: Glucagon and glicentin immunoreactivity are topographically segregated in the alpha granules of the human pancreatic A-cell. Nature 284:66, 1980

23. Ravazzola M et al.: Immunocytochemical localisation of prosomatostatin fragments in maturing and mature secretory granules of pancreatic and gastrointestinal cells. Proc Nat Acad Sci USA 80:215, 1983

24. Varndell IM et al.: Intracellular topography of immunoreactive gastrin demonstrated using electron immunocytochemistry. Experientia 39, 713–717, 1983

24a. Marangos PJ, Zis AP, Clark RI, et al.: Neuronal, non-neuronal and hybrid forms of enolase in brain: structural, immunological and functional comparison. Brain Res 150:117–133, 1978

24b. Carlei F, Polak JM: Antibodies to neuron specific enolase for the delineation of the entire diffuse neuroendocrine system in health and disease. Semin Diagn Pathol 1:59, 1983

25. Moore BW: A soluble protein characteristic of the nervous system. Biochem Biophys Res Commun 19:739–744, 1965

26. Ferri G-L, Probert L, Cocchia D, et al.: Evidence for the presence of S-100 protein in the glial component of the human enteric nervous system. Nature 297:409–410, 1982

27. Hobbs SE, Polak JM: Quantitative immunocytochemistry. In: Gut Hormones, 1st edition. SR Bloom, ed. Edinburgh, Churchill Livingstone, 1978, p 87–91

28. Solcia E, Capella C, Vassallo G: Endocrine cells of the stomach and pancreas in states of gastric hypersecretion. R C Gastronterol (Rome) 2:147, 1970

29. Solcia E, Capella C, Vassallo G, et al.: Endocrine cells of the gastric mucosa. Int Rev Cytol 42:223, 1975

30. Solcia E, Capella C, Buffa R, et al.: Pathology of the Zollinger-Ellison syndrome. In: Progress in Surgical Pathology, vol. 1. New York, Masson, 1980, p. 119

31. Creutzfeldt W, Arnold R, Creutzfeldt C, et al.: Gastrin and G-cells in the antral mucosa of patients with pernicious anaemia, acromegaly and hyperparathyroidism and in a Zollinger-Ellison tumour of the pancreas. Europ J Clin Invest 1:461, 1971

32. Solcia E, Frigerio B, Capella C: Gastrin and related endocrine cells modulating gastric secretion. In: Gastrins and the vagus, JF Rehfeld and E Amdrup, Eds. London, Academic Press, 1979, p. 31

33. Pearse AGE, Polak JM, Bloom SR, et al.: The newer gut hormones; cellular sources, physiology, pathology and clinical aspects. Gastroenterology 72:746,1977

34. Zollinger RM: The ulcerogenic (Zollinger-Ellison) syndrome. In: Surgical endocrinology, SR Friesen, ed. Philadelphia, J.B. Lippincott, 1978

35. Bhagavan BS, Hofkin GA, Woel GM, et al.: Zollinger-Ellison syndrome: Ultrastructural and histochemical observations in a child with endocrine tumorlets of gastric antrum. Arch Path 98:217, 1974

36. Russo A, Buffa R, Grasso G, et al.: Gastric gastrinoma and diffuse G-cell hyperplasia associated with chronic atrophic gastritis. Endoscopic detection and removal. Digestion 20:416, 1980
37. Royston CMS, Brew DSJ, Garnham JR, et al.: The Zollinger-Ellison syndrome due to an infiltrating tumour of the stomach. Gut 13:638, 1972
38. Hansky J: Gastrin in duodenal ulcer disease. In: Gastrin and the vagus. Ed. JF Rehfeld and E Amdrup, London, Academic Press, 1979, p. 273
39. Solcia E, Capella C, Buffa R, et al.: Endocrine cells of the gastrointestinal tract and related tumours. Pathobiol Annu 9:163, 1979
40. Sjolund K, Alumets J, Berg N-O, et al.: Duodenal endocrine cells in adult coeliac disease. Gut 20:547, 1979
40a. Ratzenhofer M, Aubock L, Becker H: Elektronen- und fluoreszenz-mikroskopische Untersuchungen der Appendicit neurogene. Verh Dtsch Ges Path 53:218, 1969
41. Sipple JH: The association of pheochromocytoma with carcinoma of the thyroid gland. Am J Med 31:163, 1961
42. Wermer P: Genetic aspects of adenomatosis of endocrine glands. Am J Med 16:363, 1954
43. Gould VE, Chejfec G: Neuroendocrine carcinomas of the colon. Ultrastructural and biochemical evidence of their secretory function. Am J Surg Pathol 2:31, 1978
44. Balls KF, Nicholson JTL, Goodman HL, et al.: Functional islet cell carcinomas of the pancreas with Cushing's syndrome. J Clin Endocrinol 19:1134, 1959
45. Larsson LI, Grimelius L, Hakanson R, et al.: Mixed endocrine pancreatic tumours producing several peptide hormones. Am J Pathol 79:271, 1975
46. Polak JM, Adrian TE, Bryant MG, et al.: Pancreatic polypeptide in insulinomas, gastrinomas, vipomas, glucagonomas. Lancet i:328, 1977
47. Creutzfeldt W: Pancreatic endocrine tumours—the riddle of their origin and hormone secretion. In: Contemporary topics in the study of diabetes and metabolic endocrinology. Ed. SHA Shafrir, New York, Academic Press, 1974
48. Solcia E, Capella C, Buffa R, et al.: Morphological and functional classifications of endocrine cells and related growths in the gastrointestinal tract. In: Gastrointestinal hormones. GBJ Glass, ed. New York, Raven Press, 1980
49. Mallinson CN, Bloom SR, Warin AP, et al.: A glucagonoma syndrome. Lancet 2:1, 1974
50. Mallinson CN, Bloom SR: The hyperglycemic, cutaneous syndrome: pancreatic glucagonoma. In: Surgical endocrinology, clinical syndromes. Friesen SR, ed. Philadelphia, J.B. Lippincott, 1978
51. Rehfeld JF, Stadil F, Malmstrom J, et al.: Gastrin heterogeneity in serum and tissue: a progress report. In: Gastrointestinal hormones, Thompson J, ed. Austin, Univers Texas Press, 1975
52. Rehfeld JF, Schwartz TW, Stadil F: Immunochemical studies on macromolecular gastrin: evidence that "Big big gastrin" are artifacts in blood and mucosa, but truly present in some large gastrinoma. Gastroenterology 73:469, 1977
53. Broder LE, Carter SK: Pancreatic islet cell carcinoma. Clinical features of 52 patients. Ann Intern Med 79:101, 1973
54. Larsson LI, Holst JJ, Kuhl C, et al.: Pancreatic somatostatinoma: clinical features and physiological implications. Lancet i:666–668, 1977
54a. Zollinger RM, Ellison EH: Primary peptic ulcerations of the jejunum associated with islet cell tumours of the pancreas. Ann Surg 142:709, 1955
55. Walsh JH, Grossman MI: Gastrin. N Engl J Med 292:1324, 1975
56. Speranza V, Basso N, Lezoche E: Effects of bombesin and calcium on serum gastrin

levels in patients with retained or excluded antral mucosa. In: Gastrointestinal hormones and pathology of the digestive system. MI Grossman, V Speranza, N Basso, E Lezoche, eds. New York, Plenum Press, 1978, p. 319–324

57. Marks C: Carcinoid tumours: A clinicopathological study. Marks C, ed. Boston, GK Hall, 1979

58. Solcia E, Capella, C, Vassallo G: Lead-haematoxylin as a stain for endocrine cells. Significance of staining and comparison with other selective methods. Histochemie 20:116, 1969

59. Kohler G, Milstein C: Continuous cultures of fused cells secreting antibody of pre-defined specificity. Nature 256:495, 1975

60. Tapia FJ, Barbosa AJA, Marangos PJ, et al.: Neuron specific enolase is produced by neuroendocrine tumours. Lancet ii:808, 1981

61. Passaro E Jr: Current concepts in diagnosis. In: Surgical endocrinology: clinical syndromes. Friesen SR, ed. Philadelphia, J.B. Lippincott, 1978

62. Larsson LI, Rehfeld JF, Sundler F, et al.: Pancreatic gastric in foetal and neonatal rats. Nature 262:609, 1976

63. Hoffman JW, Fox PS, Milwaukee SDW: Duodenal wall tumours and the Zollinger-Ellison syndrome. Arch Surg 107:334, 1973

64. Creutzfeldt W: Endocrine tumours of the pancreas. In: The diabetic pancreas. Wellman KF and Volk BW, eds. Plenum Press, New York, p. 551, 1977

64a. Larsson LI: ACTH-like immunoreactivity in the gastrin cell. Independent changes in gastrin and ACTH-like immunoreactivity during ontogeny. Histochemistry 56:245, 1978

65. Stefanini P, Carboni M, Patrassi N, et al.: Beta islet cell tumors of the pancreas. Results of a study on 1,067 cases. Surgery 75:597, 1974

66. Creutzfeldt S, Arnold R, Creutzfeldt C, et al.: Biochemical and morphological investigations of 30 human insulinomas. Diabetologia 9:217, 1973

67. Fiocca R, Capella C, Buffa R, et al.: Glucagon-, glicentin- and pancreatic polypeptide-like immunoreactivities in rectal carcinoids and related colorectal cells. Am J Path 100:81, 1980

68. Warner TFCS, Block M, Reza Mafez G, et al.: Glucagonomas. Ultrastructure and immunocytochemistry. Cancer 51:1091–1096, 1983

69. Grimelius L, Hultquist GT, Stenkvist B: Cytological differentiation of asymptomatic pancreatic islet cell tumours in autopsy material. Virchows Arch A 365:275, 1975

70. Bloom SR, Polak JM: Glucagonomas, VIPomas and PPomas. 1979. In: Gut Peptides, Miyoshi A, ed. Kodansha, Tokyo

71. Said SI, Faloona GR: Elevated plasma and tissue levels of vasoactive intestinal polypeptide in the watery-diarrhea syndrome due to pancreatic, bronchogenic and other tumours. New Engl J Med 293:155, 1975

71a. Bloom SR, Christophides MD, Tatemoto K, et al.: All vipomas produce PHI. Regulatory Peptides 6:30, 1983

72. Tatemoto K, Mutt V: Isolation of two novel candidate hormones using a chemical method for finding naturally occurring polypeptides. Nature 285:417–418, 1980

73. Bloom SR, Christofides ND, Delamarter J et al.: Tumour coproduction of VIP and PHI explained by single coding gene. Lancet ii:1163–1165, 1983

74. Itoh N, Obata K-I, Yanihara N et al.: Human preprovasoactive intestinal polypeptide contains a novel PHI-27-like peptide, PHM-27. Nature 304:547–548, 1983

75. Blackburn AM, Bryant MG, Adrian TE, Bloom SR: Pancreatic tumours produce neurotensin. J Clin Endocrinol Metab 52:820–822, 1981

76. Bloom SR, Lee YC, Lacroute JM, et al: Two patients with pancreatic apudomas secreting neurotensin and VIP. In press in Gut.
77. Frohman LA, Zabo M, Berelowitz M, Stachura ME: Partial purification and characterization of a peptide with GH releasing activity from extra pituitary tumours in patients with acromegaly. J Clin Invest 65:43–55, 1980
78. Guillemin R, Brazeau P, Bohlen P, et al.: Growth hormone releasing factor from a human pancreatic tumour that caused acromegaly. Science 218:585–587, 1982
79. Rivier J, Spiess J, Thorner, M, Vale W: Characterization of a growth hormone releasing factor from a human pancreatic islet. Nature 300:276–278, 1982
79a. Bensch KG, Gordon GB, Miller LR: Studies on the bronchial counterpart of the Kultzchitzky (argentaffin) cell and innervation of bronchial glands. J Ultrastruc Res 12:668–686, 1965
80. Vale W, Brazeau P, Rivier C, et al.: Somatostatin. Rec Progr Horm Res 34:365, 1975
80a. Kahn CR, Bhathena SJ, Recant L, et al.: Use of somatostatin and somatostatin analogs in a patient with a glucagonoma. J Clin Endocrinol Met 53:543–549, 1981
81. Long RG, Peters JR, Bloom SR, et al.: Somatostatin, gastrointestinal peptides and the carcinoid syndrome. Gut 22:549, 1981
82. Craig RK, Hall L.: Recombinant DNA technology: application to the characterization and expression of polypeptide hormones. In: Genetic Engineering, Williamson R, ed. New York, Academic Press, 1983

# 2 | Zollinger–Ellison Syndrome—Current Issues

*Denis M. McCarthy*
*Robert T. Jensen*

## INTRODUCTION

Zollinger–Ellison syndrome (ZES) is characterized by persistent basal gastric hyperacidity due to hypergastrinemia of tumor origin. Over the past decade its diagnosis and management have been much discussed, in contrast to previously when opinion was uniformly in favor of and management by total gastrectomy. This article addresses principally those areas in which change has been appreciable and does not deal with history, pathology, pathogenesis, clinical features, or results of classical surgical therapy; these are mostly well known and have been reviewed in detail elsewhere.[1-8] Rather, it addresses the impact of identification of different clinical subgroups whose disease may not be identical, of changing diagnostic methodology and increased ability to find and excise tumors, and of the employment of newer medical and surgical approaches to management. In addition, it identifies some deficiencies in current knowledge which limit our ability to take care of patients optimally. Finally, it offers some insights into why medical therapy for the condition has not succeeded in all cases.

## ALTERED SETTING OF ILLNESS

In the past, ZES was usually diagnosed late in the condition and only in the context of multiple or ectopic ulcers and fulminant ulcer disease. Nowadays, most cases have a 3-to-5-year history of relatively typical duodenal ulcer disease,

25

are mostly diagnosed before the first operative intervention, and in 18–25 percent of cases have no ulcer detectable at the time of diagnosis.[6] Surgical mortality surrounding total gastrectomy is much reduced, and need for operation has also declined considerably. Anastomotic ulcer or other complications of previous gastric surgery are less frequent presentations, but severe esophageal disease due to ZES is increasingly recognized.[9] When ulcer disease resistant to newer antiulcer drugs, e.g., Cimetidine, Ranitidine, Sucralfate, etc., is encountered, patients usually have a serum gastrin determination and, if elevated, acid secretory studies. Thus, failure of conventional therapy for duodenal ulcer is another setting in which the disease may present. Death from fulminant peptic ulcer disease or its attendant complications is nowadays rarely seen; death from tumor progression is the rule. Whether or not early diagnosis and newer forms of treatment have lowered mortality has not been established in a controlled setting, but among investigators it is widely believed that survival has been prolonged, and that overall mortality has been reduced.

Beyond clinical ZES, it is increasingly recognized that the syndrome can exist in subclinical forms, particularly in patients or kindreds with multiple endocrine neoplasia—Type I (MEN-I). There is no generally accepted procedure for screening such subjects. Even where specific tests are employed as distinct from "family history," there is no agreement as to the best types of tests, the frequency at which they should be performed or repeated, or the procedure to be followed when positive tests are encountered in asymptomatic subjects. As will be seen below, the data base is simply not adequate to answer all of these currently important questions. There is an urgent need for investigators to cooperate more in the systematic collection and pooling of such data so that ten years from now our management decisions will be less empirical.

## PATIENT SUBGROUPS IN ZES

In the era of total gastrectomy, all patients with hypergastrinemic, hypersecretory disorders, presumed or demonstrated due to tumor, were grouped together, since treatment was similar in all. As a result, most of the published literature affecting pathology, diagnosis, treatment, outcome, and natural history of ZES has failed to separate patients with "sporadic" ZES from those whose tumors occur as part of the MEN-I syndrome. As a result of this, we have little information on the pathology, diagnosis, and management of ZES in MEN-I specifically. Increasing evidence points to the conclusion that the problems posed by MEN-I are not identical to those attending "sporadic" ZES. The pathology of these conditions has recently been reviewed[2,8] and will not be dealt with here except as it affects clinical management. In various series,[8] it appears that in about two-thirds of ZES patients, gastrinomas are "sporadic," lacking any family history, and in one-third are "genetic," having other features of MEN-I. They generally, but not invariably, have a positive family history of some feature of the MEN-I trait other than ulcer disease. Most non-pancreatic gastrinomas are "sporadic" although they constitute only a minority of sporadic tumors. On the other hand, most tumors in MEN-I patients are found in the pancreas or exceptionally in the duodenal wall. According to Friesen,[10] "antral-G-cell-hyperplasia" (AGCH) (diagnostic criteria unclear) is also part of the MEN-I syndrome, but few if any AGCH patients have the degree of acid hypersecretion likely to be confused with ZES. Most of the sporadic tumors are solitary, malignant, and usually found in older subjects. On the other hand, tumors in MEN-I are generally small, multiple, "benign," and mostly seen for the most part in younger subjects, who may or may not have overt ZES. With prolonged observation some MEN-I tumors prove metastatic, but the frequency or nature of this transition is unclear. The incidence of metastases has not been examined in the two groups matched for age. It is possible that by the time MEN-I patients reach the age at which most sporadic tumors occur (fifth to eights decades) the incidence of malignancy is similar in both groups. However, the multicentric nature of the tumors in MEN-I suggests that the diseases are separate and not merely different phenotypic manifestations of the same genetic trait.

Sporadic gastrinomas generally occur in the pancreas, though primary tumors also occur not uncommonly in the walls of the stomach, duodenum or jejunum,[2,8] with duodenal wall tumors accounting for 6–23 percent of primary tumors found at surgery.[6,7] Since the adult human pancreas has no gastrin-containing cells (G-cells) and since these cells occur normally in stomach, duodenum, and jejunum, pancreatic tumors are generally considered "ectopic," while the latter three sites give rise to "entopic" tumors. The incidence of malignant change seems much higher (60–70 percent) in ectopic than in entopic (38 percent) tumors,[11] and excision of duodenal wall tumors carries about a 50 percent chance of cure.[3,4]

Ectopic primary tumors also occur in lymph glands,[2,3,12–14] in the splenic hilum, root of the mesentery, omentum, liver, gall bladder, ovary and parathyroid.[8] Unless a primary tumor has already been identified, solitary tumors in these sites should not be regarded as metastases since excision may cure the patient. The cure rate for excision of solitary, non-pancreatic ectopic tumors is unknown, due to the rarity of such lesions. However, the probability of a surgeon finding a primary tumor in the pancreas has rarely exceeded 50 percent, and it seems increasingly likely that the occurrence of primary tumors in unexpected locations has contributed significantly to operative and preoperative failures to find them.

The MEN-I syndrome accounts for about one-third of all cases of ZES, the latter occurring in 52–61 percent of affected MEN-I subjects.[10,15,16] Over 90 percent of MEN-I patients develop hyperparathyroidism,[10,16] and only following this development does ZES become detectable by current screening tests.[17] This sequence in no way excludes the possibility raised by Vance and colleagues[18-20] that the hyperparathyroidism (usually hyperplasia of all four glands) is secondary to the presence of a pancreatic tumor. When hypercalcemia develops, it exacerbates subclinical ZES and facilitates detection. In the 10 percent of MEN-I patients who do not have hyperparathyroidism and hypercalcemia, it is possible that the combination of rapid calcium infusion followed by a secretin provocation test would unmask very early cases of ZES not detectable by secretin provocation alone. One recent test has employed this kind of calcium-secretin provocation with good results, but whether this was in MEN-I patients or in sporadic cases or both was not stated.[21] Suffice it to say, normocalcemic MEN-I patients with intact parathyroid glands are unlikely to have fasting hypergastrinemia or to respond to secretin provocation tests.[16,17] This may hamper detection of subclinical gastrinoma in such cases.

The multiplicity and small size of pancreatic tumors found in MEN-I cause difficulties in finding the tumors preoperatively or in justifying laparotomy as an additional diagnostic step, even though the tumors appear benign for much of the patient's life span. On theoretical grounds, one could make a case for radical pancreatico-duodenectomy in young MEN-I patients, but most surgeons feel that the mortality and morbidity associated with this would be unacceptably high.

At the present time, most authorities do not accept pancreatic islet hyperplasia or nesidioblastosis as causes of ZES though they may be found in MEN-I patients with gastrinoma.[8,22] "Antral G-cell hyperplasia" may be associated with hypergastrinemia, duodenal ulcers, and mild increases in acid output. All three conditions, therefore, may occur in MEN-I, but there is no solid evidence that they ever cause an illness resembling ZES. The finding of islet cell hyperplasia or nesidioblastosis should not be used to justify removal of part or all of the pancreas.

## DIAGNOSIS

Diagnostic assessment of ZES involves four basic issues: (1) identification of the secretory diathesis; (2) documentation of the nature and extent of the associated acid-peptic disease; (3) location of the primary tumor(s); and (4) assessment for malignant versus benign disease. In the majority of patients, ZES presents in the fifth through eighth decades of life; careful overall evaluation may reveal the existence of significant disease in other systems (e.g., cardiac, pulmonary, renal, etc.), which may have an important bearing on ZES management in that patient. If the diagnosis is confirmed, all first-degree relatives and their offspring should be placed under long-term surveillance. In MEN-I kindreds, screening should include a serum calcium, serum gastrin, and a secretin test, and screening should be repeated at least every five years even in asymptomatic cases. Recent studies suggest that serum concentrations of human pancreatic polypeptide (hPP) are of value in following MEN-I but not sporadic ZES subjects, for the development of gastrinoma or other endocrine, pancreatic tumors.[23] Elevation of serum (hPP) seems to be a sensitive and fairly specific marker for the occurrence (or recurrence) of both functional and nonfunctional pancreatic endocrine tumors, provided that age-matched controls are employed and that only large elevations in analytical/control ratios are pursued diagnostically.[23]

### Identification of Hypersecretory Disorder

The essential feature of ZES is gross hypersecretion of gastric acid. Without evidence that acid secretion is markedly increased, interpretation of serum gastrin is rarely possible. The most important acid measurement is that of basal acid output (BAO); measurement of maximal acid output (MAO), peak acid output

(PAO), or various ratios—BAO/MAO, BAO/PAO—add little of discriminative value, and ratios are often misleading when BAO is not elevated. Gastric emptying of both liquids[24] and solids[25] is markedly increased in ZES. Therefore, in collecting acid, the method of Hector[26] should be employed using continuous manual suction, while the patient is lying on their left side in the Trendelenberg position. Intermittent suction, patients lying flat, on their right side, sitting at 45°, or tube placement in the antrum or pyloric channel may lead to lower and less accurate estimates of BAO.[7,26] The diagnostic level of BAO above which false positive diagnoses of ZES are minimized, is >15 mEq/h in the intact patient or >5 mEq/h in those who have had previous gastric surgery.

It should be stressed that most patients with true ZES have values for BAO between 25 mEq/h and 100 mEq/h, and most operated patients with ZES will postoperatively exceed the 15 mEq/h criteria used for intact patients. While there are reports in the literature[6] of patients recorded as having a BAO value between 10 and 15 mEq/h, who were subsequently shown to have gastrinoma, these are uncommon, and adequacy of the methodology used in collecting and titrating the gastric contents in those cases has not been established. Close attention to acid output (BAO) will avoid most of the pitfalls associated with the not uncommon false positive diagnosis of ZES. False negative diagnoses of ZES, as distinct from failures to investigate, are uncommon. Since acid secretory studies are infrequently and often poorly performed in many hospitals, clinicians have tended to place excessive reliance on the results of measurements of serum gastrin in diagnosing ZES. However, only the inappropriate elevation of serum gastrin in the hyperacidic patient should lead to investigation for ZES.

In the event that satisfactory gastric juice samples for analysis can not be obtained, measurement of serum group I pepsinogens by radioimmunoassay (RIA) is extremely helpful in interpreting hypergastrinemia. The normal range for Group I pepsinogens is 20–100 ng/ml. A value <20 ng/ml is invariably associated with absent or very low acid output.[27-29] Values >100 ng/ml are associated with hypersecretion, irrespective of etiology. Patients with ZES may exceed 250 ng/ml, but up to one-fourth of duodenal ulcer patients have values in the ZES range.[27] Hyperpepsinogenemia-I has the same significance as an elevated BAO. Its presence excludes the possibility that hypergastrinemia is due to hypochlorhydria, but the lower limit of the test, below which the diagnosis of ZES should be considered very unlikely, has not been determined precisely.

In spite of widespread availability of serum gastrin determinations, the accuracy of such tests remains poor in many hospitals. Both intra- and interassay variation may be unacceptably high, and normal ranges differ a lot from laboratory to laboratory. For this reason, each laboratory must determine its own range of normal values and its own sense of the range of values encountered in relevant disease controls (i.e., truncal vagotomy, billroth-II gastrojejunostomy, duodenal ulcer). In like manner, the laboratory must inform clinicians as to the range over which sample concentrations are linear, the range of variation of repeated basal samples, the increment which constitutes a significant increase over baseline following secretin injection, and whether or not other common substances, such as heparin, interfer with the results. If detailed information of this kind is not available, then the clinician should send all the relevant samples from the patient to an established reference laboratory. All samples from a timed test should be analyzed in the same assay, after careful collection and processing according to the methods recommended by that laboratory.

If acid secretory rate (BAO) and fasting serum gastrin (FSG) are not measured with close attention to detail, then the criteria listed here are of little value. FSG rises somewhat with age so that in many cases being investigated for ZES, age-matched normal patient values will lie towards the upper limit of the assay range (mean + 2 S.D.). Only values which exceed the age-matched range merit serious investigation for ZES, unless the BAO is very high and the patient has clinical features of the disease. The majority of true ZES patients have an FSG >1000 pg/ml and most exceed 500 mg/ml; values between 200 pg/ml and 500 pg/nl, while suspect, are usually not due to ZES. These crude figures serve only as rough guidelines, and more precise figures must be developed by the investigating laboratory (and not by the manufacturer of the assay kit).

If FSG and BAO are simultaneously elevated, investigation for ZES should proceed to performance of a secretin test. This test has recently been reviewed in detail by McGuigan and Wolfe[30] and by Lamers.[31] The patient, after two basal FSG determinations, is given an I.V. bolus injection of 2 iu/kg GIH secretin (Pharmacia, Inc.). Blood is drawn for serum gastrin determinations at 2, 5, 10, 15, and 30 minutes post injection and a response curve drawn as shown in Figure 2-1. An increment in peak serum gastrin, of >200 pg/ml above mean basal, estab-

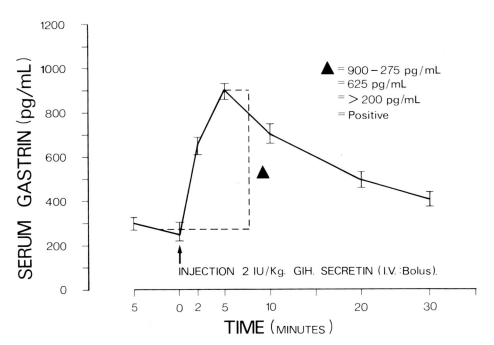

**Fig. 2-1.**   Response to a secretin (bolus) test in a patient with ZES.

lishes the diagnosis provided that the antibody used in the assay recognizes G-17 and G-34 gastrins equally. If all of these conditions are met, false positive diagnoses are extremely rare and false negative tests uncommon (10–15 percent). False negative tests may be caused by hypocalcemia,[32] and one recent paper advocates combining the secretin bolus test routinely with rapid calcium loading.[21] Secretin tests employing I.V. infusions, other doses, or other proprietary preparations of secretin, other antigastrin antibodies, or other criteria for positivity,[8] cannot be evaluated at this time. Secretin tests are not meaningful in hypochlorhydric or achlorhydric patients and are probably unnecessary when FSG exceeds 1000 pg/ml. Because tumors have been found in patients with allegedly negative secretin tests, a positive test cannot be regarded as essential to establishing the diagnosis. However, a negative secretin test casts sufficient doubt on the diagnosis, that total gastrectomy should not be performed without histologic proof of the presence of tumor. False positive tests are similarly hard to evaluate. A laparotomy which fails to find a tumor may be missing adenomas which are present but are either small in size or ectopic in location. There are some very rare cases in which false positive tests may have occurred in people later cured by antrectomy.[33] There is also a lack of adequate data on the responses to I.V. bolus secretin injections in relevant disease controls (antral hyperfunction, isolated retained antrum, chronic gastric outlet obstruction, proximal Crohn's disease, post-vagotomy and diabetic gastroparesis, etc.). Nevertheless, a clearly positive response, as in Figure 2-1, is strong evidence for the existence of gastrinoma. No other provocative test is of established value in ZES.

## Documentation of the Extent of Acid-Peptic Disease: Endoscopy

Most of the structural injuries caused by ZES are in the upper GI tract. The most useful procedure for assessing their severity is upper GI endoscopy. The esophagus may be the site of unexpectedly severe disease.[9] Distal esophageal disease may create serious difficulty in performing total gastrectomy and esophago-jejunostomy. Similarly, the finding of esophageal reflux or gastric outlet obstruction should make one reluctant to perform highly selective (proximal gastric) vagotomy; the operation may increase reflux and esophageal mucosal injury or may exacerbate stasis when the outlet is obstructed.

Apart from prominent gastric rugal folds and visible hypersecretion, the stomach is generally unremarkable in ZES. Gastric ulcer and gastric erosions occur occasionally but are uncommon. Gastritis, as judged by erythema and friability, is not usually apparent. Beyond the pylorus, pathological findings are almost universal. Erosive duodenitis, ulcers in the duodenal bulb, and post-bulbar ulcers and erosions, with jejunal ulcerations at times are all encountered. Nowadays most people with ZES have typical though often multiple duodenal ulcers. Jejunal ulcers have become quite uncommon. Small tumors or other lesions distal to the bulb may be hard to find due to hypermotility, copious secretions, and prominent mucosal folds. Occasionally, a primary tumor occurs in gastric mucosa or in the duodenal wall; small tumors may easily be missed in either of these sites, unless appropriate medication is employed during endoscopy. When the diagnosis is known before the procedure, the patient's normal dose of medications should be given orally about 1 hour prior to endoscopy (e.g., Cimetidine 300–600 mg plus 10 mg isopropamide). However, if the clinician suspects for the first time the diagnosis of ZES during endoscopy, he should give the patient intravenous Cimetidine (300–600 mg by intravenous infusion over 10 minutes) and parenteral anticholinergic therapy (glycopyrrolate 0.1 mg I.M. or I.V., repeated after 5 minutes if necessary). When the scope is in the duodenum, 1 mg of glucagon may be injected I.V. and repeated in 3–5 minutes if motility returns. The duodenum should be inflated rapidly, effacing folds as much as possible, so that any focal abnormalities (ulcers, tumors, etc.) can be visualized and biopsied. If this approach fails, a side-viewing endoscope should be employed. Careful examination of the duodenal wall is most important, as endoscopy has resulted in location and removal of duodenal primary tumors in a number of cases.[34-36] Up to 20 percent of detectable tumors may be found in the duodenal wall.[3,4,8,37]

Endoscopy is also important in the long-term care of the patient. Since ulcers and erosions may come and go rapidly, drawings of lesions should be made and their exact positions recorded so that on re-endoscopy development of new lesions can be differentiated from persistence of old ones. This is of importance in evaluating the adequacy of drug therapy.

## Location of Primary Tumors

The attainment of an ideal management strategy for ZES continues to be limited by the practical difficulty of finding the gastrinoma(s) causing the syndrome in 20–60 percent of cases. Simpler tests, such as barium meal, air contrast radiography, hypotonic duodenography, or upper gastrointestinal endoscopy, may rarely (<10 percent of cases) lead to detection of the primary tumor; while these are worth doing, no reliability can be placed on a negative outcome of any such test. Selective angiography, a technique quite useful in visualizing insulinoma, glucagonoma, and Werner-Morrison non-$\beta$ islet cell adenomas, to date has been less useful in ZES. It achieves visualization of the primary tumor in only a minority of cases[38-40] but often is of great value in demonstrating hepatic metastases not easily detected by other techniques. Angiographic studies should always start with selective injection of the hepatic artery. If metastases are present, information on the size and location of the primary tumor is less important, but may still be worthwhile in some patients (see below). While CT-scanning[41] and ultrasonic scanning[42,43] are probably better than angiography, both have considerable shortcomings. At times angiography, CT-scanning, and ultrasound may be complimentary; at other times more than one of the imaging techniques is "positive" though their predictions contradict each other as to the location of the tumor within the pancreas.[8] Furthermore, many functionally significant, resectable, benign tumors are at or below the limits of resolution of the techniques. CT scan results may be improved by infusion of cholegrafin contrast medium,[6] but the x-ray absorption coefficient of tumor tissue does not differ much from that of surrounding tissues, and ultrasonic scanning has proved superior in two studies.[42,43] The latter modality has a number of advantages; it is noninvasive, inexpensive, and devoid of radiation hazard, but its performance and interpretation require considerable operator skill. When all these tests are combined, not more than 40–50 percent of tumors are confidently identified prior to exploration. Until recently surgical exploration did not appear to add much to preoperative localization, except when tumors were in the duodenal wall or in ectopic locations. The comparative value of such tests has not been studied systematically in the same ZES population.

Two other recently introduced techniques offer some hope of improved ability to localize tumor. The more studied, though so far only in small groups of patients,[6,44-49] is percutaneous transhepatic portal venous sampling (PTPVS). In this technique, steerable catheters are introduced through the right chest wall into the liver and guided into hepatic branches of the portal vein, and thence in retrograde fashion into portal vein tributaries (e.g., splenic, superior mesenteric), which receive the venous drainage of the pancreas. Such veins can be sampled and their gastrin content measured. Venography is performed at the same time so that the vein being sampled can be identified and relocated. Ideally, one hopes to find a single vein with a large increment (>1000 pg/ml) in serum gastrin, when concentration in the vein is compared to that in the systemic circulation or in the portal vein. However, not uncommonly much smaller gradients are found in more than one vein simultaneously, with patterns of distribution of concentration of gastrin that are at best accurate but hard to explain and, at worst, the result of any of a number of sampling artifacts. In addition to difficulties with interpretation in many cases, the technique is costly, requires great expertise, time, and effort on the part of the angiographer, and considerable endurance powers on the part of the patient. Undoubtedly, a number of tumors have been detected by this method, but it is not clear from published reports that the tumors in these cases could not be detected by other methods, or that the test predictions correlated closely with operative findings and reduced the time taken to find the tumor. One would also have liked to ask the surgeon if he could have found the same tumor without PTPVS. False negative results are not uncommon.[47,49]

Preliminary results suggest that PTPVS may aid in the management of patients with sporadic or ectopic gastrinomas (solitary tumors) but not of MEN-I patients (multiple small adenomas), who are much less likely to benefit from location and excision of tumor.[37,48] Availability of a rapid assay for gastrin, which could be used in an operative setting to check on the completeness of tumor removal, might enhance the usefulness of venous sampling; so far there are no published studies claiming success in this. Microdensitometric histochemical assays[50] may be more useful in this area than conventional radioimmunoassays which delay results. In general, the use of PTPVS seems destined to be confined to special centers.

Far more promising but much less studied is the use of intraoperative ultrasonic scanning of the exposed pancreas. This technique, developed at the University of Illinois,[51] is now being evaluated at NIH and at major medical centers in Seattle, Los Angeles, and Dallas, which have particular interests in the surgery of endocrine pancreatic tumors. Gastrinomas are relatively sonolucent. Within close range of the detector, artifacts of ultrasonic scanning are minimal and resolution appears excellent. The device is inexpensive, simple to use, and results are immediately available. Preoperative PTPVS may greatly facilitate the use of intraoperative ultrasound by identifying the area of interest in the pancreas; the surgeon can then concentrate on a defined area. The combination of PTPVS, laparotomy, and operative scanning seems at this point to have the greatest potential for accurate localization of tumors, thus facilitating curative resection; results are awaited with great interest.

Laparotomy itself has definite merit as a diagnostic approach, at least in certain patients, but it must be stressed that the kind of laparotomy required is time consuming and is not without hazard. It involves entering the lesser sac, mobilizing the spleen, the body and tail of the pancreas, the stomach, and the duodenum adjacent to the head of the pancreas. The whole area surrounding the pancreas is searched, including the omentum, the rest of the mesentery, lymph nodes, the hilum of the spleen, the gastrocolic and lienogastric ligaments, the walls of the stomach and proximal intestine, and the ovaries in the female.[8] Some surgeons palpate the duodenal wall carefully and explore it only if tumor is felt; others are more aggressive and routinely perform duodenotomy with or without operative enteroscopy. Isolated duodenal wall tumors have the best prognosis among gastrinomas[3,4] and may account for most of the curably resectable cases.[37,52] Thus, it is mandatory that great care be taken in assessing the duodenum for the presence of tumor; laparotomy should only be performed by surgeons with expertise in this area.

## Assessment for "Malignant" or "Benign" Disease

As indicated earlier, it is increasingly recognized that primary sporadic gastrinomas can occur outside of the pancreaticoduodenal area, particularly in adjacent lymph glands.[2,3,12-14] Unless there is evidence of a primary tumor within the pancreas, local nodal disease should not be regarded as evidence of metastatic spread. Nodes may be detected at laparotomy or preoperatively by means of CT scan, angiography, lymphangiography, or isotopic scanning. CT-scanning or angiography will generally demonstrate the presence of hepatic metastases. Isotopic liver scans may also be helpful when there are focal metastases. Angiography or CT-scanning may occasionally demonstrate vascular invasion and nonresectability of the tumor. The histological differentiation of benign from malignant disease is often difficult, especially on frozen sections. Only direct extension of tumor through the capsule or the finding of non-lymphoidal distant metastases (e.g., in liver, lung, or bone) justify the term "malignant." The finding of neurovascular invasion, though less reliable,[53] usually indicates the presence of malignant disease. Preoperative detection of micrometastases to the liver by morphological methods is very difficult, though liver biopsy may be indicated and useful in certain cases.

Although not widely available, serological indicators of dissemination are very helpful. While not specific to gastrinoma, high serum levels of $\alpha$- or $\beta$-hCG in a ZES patient point strongly to the tumor being malignant.[54] Elevated G17/G34 gastrin ratios in serum indicate the presence of hepatic metastases with escape of G17 directly into hepatic veins and thence into the systemic circulation.[55,56] On

linergic drugs, require repeated testing for dose adjustment, and such repeated testing poses a number of difficulties. The hypersecretory disorder in ZES is relentless: discontinuing therapy is associated with rapid return of symptoms, clinical deterioration, and both hazard and discomfort to the patient, unless high-dose antacids or continuous nasogastric suction (involving prolonged fasting) are instituted. Continuous intragastric pH monitoring, without fasting and without discontinuing drugs, has much to commend it and should be associated with greater acceptance and cooperation by the patient. It also minimizes error due to dose-to-dose variation in bioavailability of drug and reflects overall steady-state control.

As to the dose of the drug, several points should be made. First, there is no generally recommended dose of any drug in ZES; specific requirements must be documented in every case and reassessed regularly. Second, there is no such thing as a patient whose acid secretion cannot be controlled, provided that adequate doses of drug are administered. Third, many of the decisions which are currently taken are arbitrary with regard to acceptability, cost, side effects, toxicity, burden of compliance, amount of benefit, etc. We, therefore, offer some guidelines, in the full knowledge that they may not apply in individual cases.

Therapy should usually be started with Cimetidine for reasons of cost, availability, and established use. When the dose exceeds 2.4 g/d, an anticholinergic drug should be added in moderate dosage. Five studies (English language) have shown that anticholinergics potentiate the effects of $H_2$-antagonists[72-76] and that the effect is sustained long term.[76,77] Pirenzepine is probably the drug of choice,[74,75] though this remains to be clearly shown in a comparative trial. Pirenzepine is not approved for sale in the U.S.A.; alternative effective marketed drugs include isopropamide (DARBID)[73] and glycopyrrolate (ROBINUL).[72] If the dose of Cimetidine, taken together with optimal doses of an anticholinergic drug, exceeds 6.0 g/day, an uncommon event or, if the patient is male and develops gynecomastia or sexual dysfunction, or if drug toxicity becomes apparent in any patient, therapy with an alternative drug should be initiated. Alternative drugs are discussed below.

While a variety of side effects have been associated with the use of Cimetidine, their overall incidence in most conditions has been low.[78] ZES is a rare syndrome, and only a fraction of cases are at risk for dose-dependent side effects. Nevertheless, the dose of drug tends to rise with time, and in males this has been associated with the development of either breast enlargement, breast tenderness, impotence, or loss of libido in up to 50 percent of long-term, high-dose cases.[60] When patients have been switched to Ranitidine, these side effects have reversed in all cases. This improvement on Ranitidine has recently been confirmed by European investigators.[79] While other side effects of Cimetidine, such as mental confusion,[80] have occurred uncommonly and for the most part unpredictably in ZES, none have posed any recurring problem to the management of the disease. High dosage may also make compliance burdensome to the patient, and long acting compounds, such as Omeprazole, may prove useful in such cases. While Ranitidine is more potent, the dosing interval attending its use in ZES has not been systematically studied[81]; so far, in reported series (see below) it has been given either 6-hourly or 8-hourly.

Failure of medical "control" occurs in a proportion of ZES patients. The frequency of medical failures varies form 0–88 percent in different series,[6,59,82,83] depending on what various authors call a "failure of medical therapy." In the literature, the term has been used to include many patients in whom a decision to carry out total gastrectomy was taken arbitrarily under a variety of circumstances. In most, symptoms were not controlled or were hard to control on comparatively low doses of Cimetidine (i.e., under 2.4 g/d), and the physician or surgeon taking care of the patient simply decided to perform total gastrectomy, without an attempt to perform dose-response studies in the patient or to increase the dose to an adequate level. Whether this decision was motivated by considerations of cost, compliance, side effects, patient acceptability, or risk-benefit ratios, or by the simple desire to operate surgically cannot be assessed from the reports. Patients who should have been excluded from medical therapy from the start are reported in the same way as patients who met initial indications for long-term medical management and who later "failed" after many years on the drug. Criteria for failure, based on either acid-secretory rates or intragastric pH while on drug, have not been employed in most. Thus, it is difficult to assess the magnitude of the problem. "Failure" in various reported series is summarized in Table 2-1.

Among these cases, several other problems have become apparent, including prescription of inadequate doses of drug,[79] failures of patients to comply with therapy,[6,8,58] diminished bioavailability of the drug,[84] and pharmacological reductions in response to adequate doses or plasma concentrations of drug.[81,85] These problems have been discussed elsewhere,[59] and resistance to $H_2$-antagonists is discussed further below. At this point, suffice it to say that because of a lack of data on measured efficacy, agreed criteria for control, and documentation of the various reasons which culminated in "failure of medical therapy," the incidence, nature, and severity of this "failure" cannot be assessed accurately. It is apparent from Table 2-1 that centers which fail to repeat acid secretory testing on a regular basis, fail to increase doses as required, or limit the dose of Cimetidine to 2.4 g/day may expect high "failure" rates. However, whether all subjects really need the dose of Cimetidine required to reduce secretion to 10 mE q/h or less, a regimen with a low failure rate (10 percent) but a high incidence of dose-related side effects (approximately 50 percent in males), remains to be seen. The overall incidence of failure when reasonable control is employed is probably well under 25 percent. Secretory criteria predictive of good control or failure require continued study. The vast majority of ZES patients are very well controlled on doses between 2.4 g/d and 6.0 g/d of Cimetidine plus anticholinergics; exceptionally rare patients have required up to 15 g/d, on prolonged follow-up and usually on progression of their disease.

**Ranitidine.** To date, only a relatively small number of ZES patients have received long-term therapy with Ranitidine, 9 in France—follow-up 10–26 months[79]—and 13 in the U.S.A—follow-up 6–25 months.[81] A smaller number of additional patients have had a variety of acute studies aimed at obtaining pharmacological information about the drug but have not been followed for long enough to comment on clinical usefulness. However, it is already clear that Ranitidine represents a useful addition to the list of drugs pharmacologically and clinically effective in ZES.[60,64,70,79-83,86-88]

**Table 2-1.** Failure of Medical Therapy in ZES

| Study | No. | Fail (%) | Study | No. | | Fail (%) |
|---|---|---|---|---|---|---|
| CREUTZFELDT[1] | 5 | 40 | MC CARTHY[7] | 61 | | 8 |
| DEVENEY[2] | 12 | 25 | BRENNAN[8] | 26 | | 23 (8) |
| BONFILS[3] | 13 | 61 | JENSEN[9] | 39 | | 10 |
| STABILE[4] | 20 | 50 | MALAGELADA[10] | 18 | | 6 |
| DEVENEY[5] | 17 | 65 | "CURE" | | 16% | |
| MIGNON[6] | 11 | 88 | STADIL[11] | 14 | | 0 |
| | | | "CURE" | | 20% | |

Highly selective vagotomy and medical therapy (Peters[12])
19 Cases: No "failures": no dose > 3.6 g/d

References: BR = Bibliographic Reference number of reference (superscript) in Table 2-1: [1] = BR22; [2] = BR111; [3] = BR113; [4] = AM J SURG 145, 17–23, 1983; [5] = BR63; [6] = BR79; [7] = BR58; [8] = Ann Surg 196, 239–245, 1982; [9] = BR6; [10] = BR37; [11] = in "Cimetidine," Westminster Hospital Symposium, 91, 1978; [12] = BR117.

As with Cimetidine, no ZES patient is controlled on the regular dose employed in ulcer therapy. The median Ranitidine dose requirement in ZES is about 1200 mg/day,[81] rising with time as does the dose of Cimetidine, with some patients requiring 6 to 9 g/day. While the drug is 5–10 times more potent in inhibiting acid secretion in normal and in DU subjects, in ZES the relative potency of Ranitidine to Cimetidine is between 2.5 to 1 and 4 to 1,[81,86] averaging about 3 to 1.[81] Thus, 900 mg/day of Ranitidine is equivalent to about 2.7 to 3.0 g/day of Cimetidine in ZES.

Pharmacokinetics of the two drugs are very similar.[89] There is no real difference in their half-lives in plasma, but because Ranitidine is more potent than Cimetidine, its effect lasts longer. In subjects with normal secretory drive, equipotent doses have the same duration of action. This does not hold true in ZES where doses of the drugs which produce the same initial reduction in BAO (i.e., equipotent doses) are followed by a longer duration of response to Ranitidine than to Cimetidine.[81] The altered potency ratio and the differences in response time in ZES, presumably are due to the relatively much greater gastrin-mediated and lesser histamine-mediated acid secretion in ZES than in normal or DU subjects. Another factor which may contribute to the altered potency ratio is the relatively greater effect of Ranitidine in inhibiting cholinesterase.[90] This might increase cholinergic potentiation of the response to gastrin while inhibiting histamine-mediated effects on acid secretion.[91] At persent, the discrepancy in potency ratio is not understood. Responses to both drugs are potentiated by anticholinergic agents.[75]

Reports in the literature that Ranitidine had efficacy where Cimetidine did not[92] have created an erroneous impression that there is some qualitative difference between the drugs with regard to their ability to inhibit acid secretion and that there may be subtypes of $H_2$-receptors. No evidence of such difference, other than in potency, is apparent at this time. A low dose of Cimetidine has less effect than a more potent dose of Ranitidine, but increasing the dose of Cimetidine should achieve the same effect as switching to Ranitidine, and at less cost. However, should anti-androgenic side effects develop due to the increased dose of Cimetidine, it is reasonable to switch therapy to Ranitidine, which does not appear to interact with androgen receptors.[93] This is required only in those males who develop the side effects on high-dose Cimetidine. So far, no side effects due to long-term Ranitidine have been seen in ZES with doses up to 6 g/d for one year and with lower doses for over 2 years.[79,81]

The daily maintenance dose of Ranitidine required to suppress acid secretion to a predetermined endpoint is closely correlated in individual patients with the dose of Cimetidine required to produce the same effect[81] and can be described by the linear equation:

$$\text{daily dose of Ranitidine} = 0.46 \text{ dose of Cimetidine} - 0.29 \ (r = 0.95).$$

Thus, patients who require a high initial dose of Cimetidine require a comparably high dose of Ranitidine, and those who "escape" from control with low-dose Cimetidine also "escape" from equipotent, low doses of Ranitidine. In patients who become "resistant," with elevations of $ED_{50}$ for Cimetidine 5-fold to 20-fold, $ED_{50}$ for Ranitidine shows similar elevations.[81] Thus, in terms of their pharmacology, the drugs appear very similar. From preliminary studies, the same may be said of "resistance" to MK-208 (Famotidine, Merck) and is very likely to apply to the newer potent $H_2$-antagonists, BRL-5644 (Etintidine, Ortho) and Nazitidine (Lilly), currently on trial. Because histamine is only one of the agonists of acid secretion in man, there are inherent limits to the ability of $H_2$-antagonists (including Ranitidine) to block acid secretion, especially in clinical situations where the hypersecretory drive is mainly mediated by gastrin(s) or cholinergic agonists. Differences in usefulness of Ranitidine and Cimetidine are more likely to emerge from considerations of cost, compliance, dosing interval, side effects, or incidence of severe toxicity. At present, there are insufficient data from ZES patients to warrant a conclusion, other than that males with significant antiandrogenic side effects of Cimetidine can be switched to Ranitidine with resolution of their problems.[60,79] This is the only area of clinically significant side effects of long-term, high-dose Cimetidine in ZES.

## Altered Responses to $H_2$-Antagonists

Doses of $H_2$-antagonists show considerable between-patient and within-patient variation in ZES. Some patients from the start require high doses of Cimetidine or Ranitidine to achieve sufficient suppression of acid secretion. The likely explanation for this is that $H_2$-antagonists block only the direct effect of histamine on acid secretion and its ability to potentiate responses to other agonists (e.g., acetylcholine and gastrin). These latter substances can continue to act independently as agonists, and to cause mutual potentiation, even when the effect of $H_2$-antagonists is maximal. Gastrin is a very powerful secretagogue in intact man and is the main agonist in ZES. Not only does it potentiate the secretory response to histamine and cholinergic agents, but it may also possess additional modes of action (e.g., increase release of histamine from fundic mucosal stores[94] or of acetylcholine or other substances from nerve fibers). On its own, the gastrin-receptor antagonist PROGLUMIDE has little effect on acid secretion in ZES patients.[95] Its effect has not been studied in $H_2$-blocked, cholinergically-blocked patients. However, on their own anticholinergic drugs[75] and highly selective vagotomy (HSV)[96] each can reduce BAO substantially in ZES. In combination therapy, with $H_2$-antagonists, they lower the dose of $H_2$-antagonist required to produce a given acid output. Conversely, they potentiate $H_2$-antagonists, leading to greater and more prolonged gastric secretory inhibition at any given dose. These observations suggest that endogenous cholinergic potentiation of acid secretion is important in ZES. This is further supported by the observation that in ZES, hypercalcemia due to hyperparathyroidism can greatly elevate the BAO,[97] an effect readily reversed by atropine but not readily by increases in Cimetidine (personal observations, unpublished); in intact animals intravenous calcium infusions are known to increase the response to acetylcholine but not to histamine.[98] Thus, increased cholinergic drive may be an important factor in apparent "resistance" to $H_2$-antagonists.

An increase in gastrin-mediated drive would similarly diminish responses to $H_2$-antagonists. Increased stimulation of acid secretion due to gastrin and/or acetylcholine may underlie the increase in $ED_{50}$ for Cimetidine or Ranitidine seen in many "resistant" or "escaping" patients. However, there is also evidence that the dominant species of gastrin present in serum alters with hepatic involvement by the disease[55,56]; this too may increase secretory drive without a corresponding increase in total serum gastrin. Increased secretory drive, "tachyphylaxis," "decreased sensitivity of the parietal cell to $H_2$-antagonists," "increase in $ED_{50}$," "drug tolerance," and "escape," are probably all different manifestations of the same basic phenomenon. However, this phenomenon is not the sole cause of poor responses to treatment with $H_2$-antagonists in ZES.

In three carefully studied patients recently described by Zemniak et al,[84] one had diminished response to normal or even elevated plasma levels of drug, as discussed above, but the other two cases appeared to have impaired absorption of oral Cimetidine, leading to low plasma concentrations: intravenous administration of the same dose was accompanied by much higher plasma levels and effective suppression of acid output. There are many potential causes of impaired or excessively delayed absorption of orally administered drug, including mechanical factors (e.g., strictures, gastric outlet obstruction or fistulae), malabsorption accompanying ZES,[99] excessively rapid transit through the intestine, especially in subjects with gastroenterostomy and truncal vagotomy and finally, alterations consequent on the effects of strong acid on the drug. The pKa for ionization of Cimetidine, a weak base, is 7.09; reduction of the intestinal pH below the normal range (pH 6–pH 8) will result in less Cimetidine in the un-ionized, absorbable form. In normals, bioavailability of Cimetidine is superior to that of Ranitidine, but whether this holds true in problem ZES cases, such as those alluded to above, has not been studied. At present, Ranitidine therapy as distinct from an increased dose of Cimetidine does not seem to be the answer to Cimetidine "resistance."

While some patients from the start require high doses of $H_2$-antagonists, others who are initially sensitive slowly develop some "resistance" to the drugs, as manifested by increasing oral dose requirements and increasing $ED_{50}$ or $IC_{50}$. The best studied case of this type is that described by Rune[85] in 1981. As serum gastrin rose (1976—4100 pg/ml; 1979—8000 pg/ml; 1980—29,000 pg/ml) and disease progressed, the dose of Cimetidine necessary to suppress BAO to 5 mE q/h in 1980 showed a 750 percent increase over the 1976 level. This study also showed that with high enough doses of drug, resistance could be overcome. This observation has been confirmed in the case reported by Collen et al.[81]

While we do not understand the precise mechanism by which the required dose increases with time, the existence of the phenomenon is undisputed. In the average patient, the dose must be increased (or additional anticholinergic drug given) about once per year; about 1 patient in 10 requires dose increases 6-monthly. While drug requirements increase in most patients, the final controlling dose is generally lower in patients who have had highly selective or proximal gastric vagotomy[82]; in these, the dose required very rarely exceeds 3.6 g/d Cimetidine (equivalent to 1.2 g/d Ranitidine). Since these resistance phenomena are likely receptor dependent, newer drugs (i.e., benzimidazoles, e.g., Omeprazole or prostaglandin analogues), which act on post-receptor steps in acid secretion, may in time replace $H_2$-antagonists in the management of ZES.

## Newer Drugs

From an experimental point of view, we are undergoing a period of rapid change in our understanding of gastric secretion. Several agents (e.g., prostaglandins,[100] TRH[101] and Somatostatin,[102] to name but a few) are capable of arresting acid secretion in ZES subjects. However, probably the most exciting new development is that of a new class of pharmacological agents, $H^+/K^+$ ATP-ase inhibitors or "proton pump inhibitors"; the best known is Omeprazole (H-168/68), a substituted benzimidazole manufactured and developed in Sweden.[103]

This agent binds almost irreversibly to parietal cells, has a prolonged duration of action, produces profound inhibition of acid secretion, and so far shows very little human toxicity. In acute studies,[104] 6 ZES patients resistant to high doses of $H_2$-antagonists were given a single dose of 80 mg omeprazole p.o., 36 hours after the last dose of Cimetidine. BAO was reduced by 98 $\pm$ 2 percent (X $\pm$ SEM) and 83 $\pm$ 6 percent during the second and 24th hours post-dose. Since the drug is acid-labile, it is best given as an enteric-coated preparation. In five patients given a single enteric-coated daily dose of 30–90 mg, acid secretion has been reduced to <5 mM/h, one hour before the next daily dose. Ulcers and diarrhea have disappeared and no toxicity has been observed. Preliminary studies in the U.S.A. confirm these findings.[105] This drug promises to revolutionize the medical therapy of ZES. However, long-term, high-dose toxicity studies have recently shown that rats develop sustained hypergastrinemia, with plasma gastrin concentrations of about 2000 pg/ml: this leads in time to gastric EC-cell hyperplasia and to gastric carcinoid tumor formation in some animals after 2 years of therapy. While this may delay marketing of the drug it is unlikely to be of great importance in ZES patients treated with low doses of drug: such patients are already hypergastinemic and are at increased risk for the development of carcinoid tumors." Omeprazole causes little change in serum gastrin in ZES. A number of analogues of omeprazole have also been developed which are currently undergoing Phase I and Phase II trials.

## Surgery

Surgical intervention in ZES now occurs in a number of different settings. These include:

1. Total gastrectomy for relief of acid peptic disease
2. Excision of gastrinoma for "cure" of disease
3. (1) and (2) combined
4. Palliative or debulking surgery
5. Highly selective vagotomy (proximal gastric vagotomy, superselective vagotomy, parietal cell vagotomy) performed to facilitate medical therapy

**Total Gastrectomy.** Because medical therapy is not simple for patients or physicians, and since it may prove costly, restrictive, or be associated with unacceptable side effects or difficulties in compliance, a minority of surgeons continue to advocate total gastrectomy as the "definitive" treatment of ZES in all cases.[106] Of course, it is not truly definitive in that it fails to address progression of the malignant tumor, the major cause of death. This issue has been examined in detail elsewhere.[4] For the most part, the morbidity and mortality associated with total gastrectomy, while modest, prohibit its routine use in patients easily controlled by medical therapy. On the other hand, patients who cannot take oral medications, absorb the drug, or maintain good compliance for any reason, or those who "cannot be controlled" by medical therapy, should have elective total gastrectomy. When performed, the operation should be combined with a Roux-en-Y esophagojejunostomy. It must be stressed that, in the hands of physicians who are skilled in the management of ZES, the need for gastrectomy is very uncommon and will become even less common in the future when newer antisecretory agents become available.

**Excision of Gastrinoma.** Following the advent of potent drugs that control hypersecretion of acid and related diseases, attention has once more turned to the issue of truly curative excision of the neoplasms responsible for the synthesis and release of gastrin. This development has been facilitated by the availability of improved techniques for preoperative and operative localization of tumor including: CT-scanning, transhepatic portal venous sampling, high quality, real-time, preoperative ultrasonic scanning, intraoperative B-mode, gray-scale, ultrasonic scanning, and most recently nuclear magnetic resonance imaging[107] (as discussed under "Location of Primary Tumors"). Most physicians and surgeons now favor a combined medical and surgical approach to management, with location of tumor and excision whenever possible seen as the most important role of the surgeon. The study reported from the Mayo Clinic[37] exemplifies this approach and, in addition, has provided some useful insights into current issues critical to management policy.

These authors report that 44 of 53 recent patients were fit for surgery and were explored; no patient explored after 1976 required total gastrectomy. If patients with MEN-I were excluded, surgical cure rate among those explored was about 20 percent, as judged by normalization of serum gastrin postoperatively and negative secretin challenge tests. Five of the seven "cures" followed excision of a tumor in the duodenal wall, a site known to be favorable to curative excision.[3,4,8,52]

In general, these duodenal wall tumors account for 6–23 percent of all tumors found at surgery,[6,8] with about half of them free of metastases and curably resectable.[3,52] Only patients with negative secretin tests postoperatively should be regarded as "cured."

In recent years, "cure" rates reported, generally with less than 5 years follow-up, have been 3 of 27,[106] 10 of 23,[108] 2 of 7,[109] 2 of 8,[48] 7 of 44,[37] 1 of 34,[110] and 4 of 69.[111] Combining all these figures, 29 of 212 cases, or 14 percent, have appeared cured by excision of gastrinoma. Seven additional "cures" have been described[14,112] without definition of the sample size from which they were drawn. Thus, about 1 in 7 of all tumors, and 1 in 2 duodenal wall tumors seem curably resectable. Failure to find tumor has generally been associated with a good prognosis.[37,113] For the most part, the various series have grouped together MEN-I patients and those with sporadic gastrinoma. However, at least 2 centers[37,48] appear to be abandoning attempts at surgical cure in MEN-I, since these patients frequently have multiple, small benign pancreatic tumors which are hard to find and often missed at surgery. Friesen, on the other hand, advocates a more vigorous approach with repeated local excision of the endocrine tumors but not major pancreatic resections; his results are among the best in the literature.[10,23,108,114,115] Better methods of screening MEN-I patients for new or recurrent tumors, and better localization techniques for finding them at surgery, are likely to increase the validity of this approach. At present, there is a great need to examine the results of all interventions in MEN-I patients separately from those in sporadic gastrinoma. This is reviewed elsewhere.[18]

**Gastrectomy plus Excision of Tumor.**   The best survival figures in large series of patients treated surgically are found in those who had local excision of as much tumor as possible in addition to total gastrectomy.[3,4,116]

**Palliative or Debulking Surgery.**   Beyond "cure," the data of Zollinger et al[116] suggest that removal of all resectable tumor prolongs life expectancy. Thus to evaluate surgery solely in terms of cure may miss much that is of benefit to the patient. There are no studies that have systematically evaluated "debulking" surgery, though on a priori reasoning, it should help medical control and delay death, provided it is not too radical. It is apparent that man generally can survive the nutritional consequences of total gastrectomy or total pancreatectomy but not of both. There is a general movement toward local excision of endocrine tumor(s) and away from radical pancreatic surgery, because of the unacceptably high perioperative mortality and frequent long-term morbidity attending major pancreatic resections. Partial resection of the liver may also be worthwhile if metastatic disease is localized (i.e., liver biopsy shows no evident dissemination at the microscopic level).

**Highly Selective Vagotomy.**   Richardson, and co-workers in Dallas[96] in 1979 reported that ZES patients, when subjected to highly selective vagotomy (HSV), experienced a marked reduction in BAO and a subsequent reduction in the dose of $H_2$-antagonist required to control their disease. Following the initial report on three patients, two subsequent abstracts published in 1982[117] and 1983[118] gave progress reports on 11 and 19 ZES patients, respectively, treated thus and followed for several years; a detailed account of the work is soon to be published.[119] In some patients who appeared cured, there has been no subsequent use of Cimetidine. However, in most, tumor remains and serum gastrin continues to be elevated. In these patients, the dose of Cimetidine fell following vagotomy, or efficacy of suppression increased at the same dose of drug. Long-term follow-up (average 27 months; maximum 5 years) shows that most patients are controlled on 2.4 g/d or less and only 2 of 19 require higher doses (3.6 g/d). These doses are considerably lower than those reported by Jensen,[60] suggesting that vagotomy does indeed potentiate the effect of Cimetidine. None of the vagotomized patients have developed bleeding, perforation, or required re-operation.

More information is needed before one can endorse the regular use of HSV in ZES, but if confirmed, this approach could be of great importance. Objections that medical "treatment failed as often in previously vagotomized patients as in patients without previous gastric surgery,"[63] do not necessarily diminish the value of HSV in ZES. First, the "failure" in most reported cases has been defined in arbitrary ways and does not mean that the patient would not have responded to increased doses of drug. Second, the increased dose ultimately required for control appears reduced by HSV. Third, the use of HSV may have delayed high dose requirements for many years. At present, delaying radical gastric surgery for even a couple of years may carry us into a new era of potent antisecretory drugs. Currently, HSV, if proven effective, promises to be very useful in ZES patients:

1. In whom no tumor is found
2. In whom advanced disease is found
3. In whom curative surgery is attempted
4. In patients in whom medical therapy is indicated but difficult
5. In situations where diagnosis is uncertain

It must be stressed that only HSV is being considered in this role. Other types of vagotomy are generally combined with drainage procedures (e.g., gastroenterostomy) which may exacerbate the severity of ZES considerably. At present use of HSV in ZES is a research procedure. In the future, newer drugs such as omeprazole may render HSV unnecessary.

# CONCLUSION

Today, most ZES patients with sporadic gastrinoma require medical control of acid-peptic disease, and surgical intervention for attempted location and excision of tumors. Whether this also holds true for MEN-I patients is not clear at this time. Medical failures in either group require total gastrectomy with Roux-en-y anastomosis, when curative excision of tumor is not feasible. HSV is an adjunct to medical therapy in several situations, including excision of tumor. The best and safest combination of medical and surgical interventions must be individualized to the particular case. The present management is summarized in Figures 2-2 and 2-3. With the development of newer potent drugs, "treatment failures" will soon be very rare. The main risk to the patient is death from malignant disease. There is an urgent need for better oncological approaches to the management of advanced malignant disease in ZES. The condition is thankfully rare, but remains as a challenge to the skill and judgment of physician and surgeon alike.

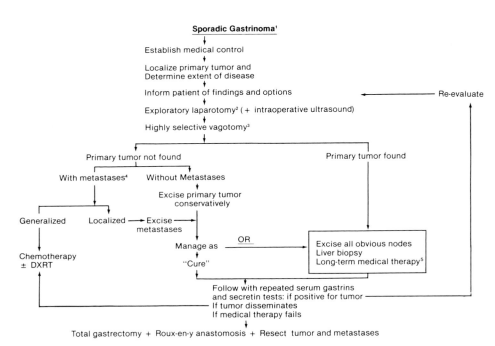

**Fig. 2-2.** Management of ZES-sporadic tumors. (1) Exclude from this figure: patients with MEN-I, patients who need or choose total gastrectomy (unsuited to medical therapy), patients totally unfit for surgery (must have medical therapy), patients in whom diagnosis is equivocal, and patients with widespread metastases detected pre-exploration. (2) Must include duodenotomy and extensive search for ectopic tumors. (3) Total gastrectomy acceptable if preoperative choice of patient: proved effective, greater morbidity and risk. (4) Patients with metastases are excluded from curative surgical excision of tumor and in need of chemotherapy: they are not excluded from medical therapy (± HSV) or total gastrectomy. (5) As outlined in text: starting with $H_2$-antagonists, adding anticholinergics, and proceeding to omeprazole, only in patients whose doses are adjusted by secretory testing or pH monitoring studies. (6) If available, G17/G34 gastrin concentration ratio or $\alpha$ or $\beta$-hCG subunit concentrations in serum may give early warning of tumor dissemination.

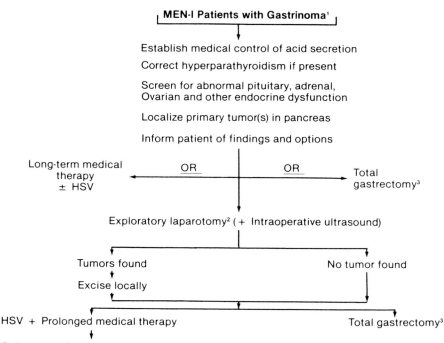

Fig. 2-3. Management of ZES in MEN-I. (1) Exclude patients with metastases, patients unsuited to medical care (need total gastrectomy), patients unsuited to total gastrectomy (must have medical therapy or medical therapy + HSV). (2) Must include duodenotomy: other ectopic sites unlikely. (3) Total gastrectomy to include also Roux-en-Y anastomosis, and excision of all resectable tumor and metastases.

# REFERENCES

1. Isenberg JI, Walsh JH, Grossman MI: Zollinger-Ellison syndrome. Gastroenterol 65:140, 1973
2. Solcia E, Capella C, Buffa R, et al: Pathology of the Zollinger-Ellison syndrome. Prog in Surg Path 1:119, 1980
3. Fox PS, Hoffman JW, DeCosse JJ, Wilson SD: The influence of total gastrectomy on survival in malignant Zollinger-Ellison tumors. Ann Surg 180:558, 1974
4. McCarthy DM: The place of surgery in the Zollinger-Ellison syndrome. N Engl J Med 302:344, and 942, 1980
5. Fang M, Ginsberg AL, Glassman L, et al: Zollinger-Ellison syndrome with diarrhea as the predominant clinical feature. Gastroenterol 76(2):378, 1979
6. Jensen RT, moderator: Zollinger-Ellison syndrome: Current concepts and management. Ann Int Med 98:59, 1983
7. McCarthy DM: Zollinger-Ellison syndrome. Annual Review of Medicine 33:197, 1982
8. McCarthy DM: The diagnosis and treatment of gastrinoma and Zollinger-Ellison syn-

drome. *In* Endocrine Related Tumors, eds. R Santen and A Manni, vol. 12 in series Cancer Treatment and Research, ed. W McGuire: Marinus Nijoff Pub., Amsterdam (in press), 1984

9. Richter JE, Pandol SJ, Castell DO, McCarthy DM: Esophageal abnormalities in the Zollinger-Ellison syndrome. Ann Int Med 95:37, 1981
10. Friesen SR: The development of endocrinopathies in the prospective screening of two families with MEA-I. World J Surg 3:753, 1979
11. Solcia E, Capello C, Buffa R, et al: Endocrine cells of the gastrointestinal tract and related tumors. Pathobiology Annual 9:163, 1979
12. Friesen SR, Bolinger RE, Pearse AGE, McGuigan JE: Serum gastrin levels in malignant Zollinger-Ellison syndrome after total gastrectomy and hypophysectomy. Ann Surg 172:504, 1970
13. Sircus W: Vagotomy in Z.E. syndrome. Gastroenterol 79:607, 1979
14. Wolfe MM, Alexander RW, McGuigan JE: Extrapancreatic, extraintestinal gastrinoma. N Engl J Med 306:1533, 1982
15. Lamers CB, Stadil F, Van Tongeren JH: Prevalence of endocrine abnormalities in patients with the Zollinger-Ellison syndrome and their families. Am J Med 64:607, 1978
16. Lamers CB, Buis JT, Van Tongeren JH: Secretin-stimulated serum gastrin levels in hyperparathyroid patients from families with multiple endocrine adenomatosis—type I. Ann Int Med 86:719, 1977
17. Betts JB, O'Malley BP, Rosenthal FD: Hyperparathyroidism: A prerequisite for Zollinger-Ellison syndrome in MEA-I: Report of a further family and a review of the literature. Quart J Med Ns XLIX, 193:69, 1980
18. Vance JE, Stoll RW, Kitabchi AE, et al: Nesiodioblastosis in familial endocrine adenomatosis. JAMA 207:1679, 1969
19. Vance JE, Stoll RW, Kitabchi AE, et al: Familial nesidioblastosis as the predominant manifestation of multiple endocrine adenomatosis. Am J Med 52:211, 1972
20. Axelrod L: Case Records of the Massachusetts General Hospital—Case 47–1974. N Engl J Med 291:1179, 1974
21. Romanus ME, Neal JA, Dilley WG, et al: Comparison of four provocative tests for the diagnosis of gastrinoma. Ann Surg 197:608, 1983
22. Creutzfeldt W, Arnold R, Creutzfeldt C, Track N: Pathomorphologic, biochemical, and diagnostic aspects of gastrinomas. Human Pathol 6:47, 1975
23. Friesen SR, Tomita T, Kimmel JR: Pancreatic polypeptide update: Its roles in detection of the trait for multiple endocrine adenopathy syndrome, type I and pancreatic polypeptide secreting tumors. Surgery 94, 5:1028, 1983
24. Dubois A, Van Eerdewegh P, Gardner JD: Gastric emptying and secretion in the Zollinger-Ellison syndrome. J Clin Invest 59:255, 1977
25. Harrison A, Ippoliti A, Cullison R: Rapid gastric emptying in Zollinger-Ellison syndrome (ZES). Gastroenterol 78:1180, 1980
26. Hector RM: Improved technique of gastric aspiration. Lancet 1:15, 1968
27. Samloff IM, Liebman WM, Panitch NM: Serum group I pepsinogens by radioimmunoassay in control subjects and patients with peptic ulcer. Gastroenterology 69:83, 1975
28. Samloff IM, Secrist DM, Passaro E Jr: A study of the relationship between serum group I pepsinogen levels and gastric acid secretion. Gastroenterol 69:1196, 1975
29. Samloff IM, Varis K, Ihamaki T, et al: Relationships among serum pepsinogen I, serum pepsinogen II, and gastric mucosal histology: A study in relatives of patients with pernicious anemia. Gastroenterol 83:204, 1982

30. McGuigan JE, Wolfe MM: Secretin injection test in the diagnosis of gastrinoma. Gastroenterol 79:1324, 1980
31. Lamers CB: Clinical usefulness of the secretin provocation test. J Clin Gastroenterol 3:255, 1981
32. Jansen JBMJ, Lamers CBHW: Effect of changes in serum calcium on secretin-stimulated serum gastrin in patients with Zollinger-Ellison syndrome. Gastroenterol 83:173, 1982
33. Primrose JN, Ratcliffe JG, Joffe SN: Assessment of the secretin provocation test in the diagnosis of gastrinoma. Brit J Surg 67:744, 1980 and correspondence, ibid, 68:217, 1981
34. Wu WC, Kengis J, Whalen GE, et al: Endoscopic localisation of a duodenal wall tumor in Zollinger-Ellison syndrome. Gastroenterol 66:1237, 1974
35. Otten MH, Bitkenhager JC, Van Blankenstein M: Zollinger-Ellison syndrome treated by endoscopic removal of a duodenal wall gastrinoma. Neth J Med 21:248, 1978
36. Donovan DC, Dureza R, Jain U: Gastrinoma of the duodenum: Diagnosis by endoscopy. NY State J Med 79:1766, 1979
37. Malagelada JR, Edis AJ, Adson MA, et al: Medical and surgical options in the management of patients with gastrinoma. Gastroenterol 84:1524, 1983
38. Giacobazzi P, Passaro E: Preoperative angiography in the Zollinger-Ellison syndrome. Ann J Surg 126:74, 1973
39. Mills SR, Doppman JL, Dunnich NR, McCarthy DM: The evaluation of angiography in Zollinger-Ellison syndrome. Radiology 131:317, 1979
40. Collen MJ, Dopman JL, Krudy AG, et al: Assessment of the ability of angiography to localise gastrinoma in patients with Zollinger-Ellison syndrome. Gastroenterol 86:1051, 1984
41. Dunnick NR, Doppman J, Mills S, McCarthy DM: Computed tomographic appearance of non-beta (or non-insulin producing) pancreatic islet cell tumors. Radiology 135:117, 1980
42. Hancke S: Localization of hormone-producing gastrointestinal tumors by ultrasonic scanning. Scand J Gastroenterol 14 (supp. 53):115, 1979
43. Shawker T, Doppman J, Dunnick NR, McCarthy DM: Ultrasonic investigation of pancreatic islet cell tumors. J Ultrasound in Medicine 1:193, 1982
44. Burcharth F, Stage JG, Stadil F, et al: Localization of gastrinomas by transhepatic portal catheterization and gastrin assay. Gastroenterol 77:444, 1979
45. Passaro E: Localization of pancreatic endocrine tumors by selective portal vein catheterization and radioimmunoassay. Gastroenterol 77:806, 1979
46. Ingemansson S: Biochemical localization of pancreaticoenteric endocrine tumors. Scand J Gastroenterol 14 (supp. 53):131, 1979
47. Feurle GE, Helmstadter V, Hoevels J, et al: Wandel von Diagnose and therapie beim Zollinger-Ellison syndrom. Dtsch Med Wschr 107:697, 1982
48. Glowniak JV, Shapiro B, Vinik AI: Percutaneous transhepatic venous sampling of gastrin. N Engl J Med 307:293, 1983
49. Cherner JA, Raufman JP, Doppman JL, et al: A prospective evaluation of percutaneous transhepatic portal venous sampling for gastrin in patients with Zollinger-Ellison syndrome (ZES). Gastroenterol 86:1046, 1984 (in press)
50. Walker W, Vinik A, Heldsinger A, Kaveh R: Role of calcium and calmodulin in activation of the oxyntic cell by histamine and carbamycholine in the guinea pig. J Clin Invest 72:955, 1983
51. Sigel B, Coelho JCU, Nyhus LM, et al: Detection of pancreatic tumors by ultrasound during surgery. Arch Surg 117:1058, 1982

52. Oberhelman HA: Excisional therapy for ulcerogenic tumors of the duodenum—long-term results. Archiv Surg 104:447, 1972
53. Bartow SA, Mukai K, Rosai J: Pseudoneoplastic proliferation of endocrine cells in pancreatic fibrosis. Cancer 47:2627, 1981
54. McCarthy DM, Weintraub B, Rosen S: Subunits of human chorionic gonadotropin in the Zollinger-Ellison syndrome. Gastroenterol 76:1198, 1979
55. Johnson JA, Fabri PJ, Lott JA: Serum gastrins in Zollinger-Ellison syndrome—identification of localized disease. Clin Chem 26:867, 1980
56. Fabri PJ, Johnson JA, Ellison EC: Prediction of progressive disease in Zollinger-Ellison syndrome—comparison of available preoperative tests. Surg Research 31:93, 1981
57. McCarthy DM, Olinger EJ, May RJ, et al: $H_2$-receptor blocking agents in the Zollinger-Ellison syndrome—experience in 7 cases and implications for long-term therapy. Ann Int Med 87:668, 1977
58. McCarthy DM: Report on the U.S. experience with Cimetidine in Zollinger-Ellison syndrome and other hypersecretory states. Gastroenterol 74:453, 1978
59. Jensen RT: Basis for failure of Cimetidine in patients with Zollinger-Ellison syndrome. Dig Dis and Sciences (editorial) 29:363, 1984
60. Jensen RT, Collen MJ, Pandol SJ, et al: Cimetidine-induced impotence and breast changes in patients with gastric hypersecretory states. N Engl J Med 308:883, 1983
61. Raufman JP, Collins SM, Pandol SJ, et al: Reliability of symptoms in assessing control of gastric acid secretion in patients with Zollinger-Ellison syndrome. Gastroenterol 84:108, 1983
62. Passaro EP, Stabile BE: Of gastrinomas and their management. Gastroenterol 84:1621, 1983
63. Deveney C, Steins S, Way LW: Cimetidine in the treatment of Zollinger-Ellison syndrome. Am J Surg 146:116, 1983
64. Mignon M, Vallot T, Mayeur S, et al: Respective influence on 24-hour gastric acidity of Cimetidine and Ranitidine in 6 cases of Zollinger-Ellison syndrome (ZES). Gastroenterol 80:1232, 1981
65. Peterson WL, Barnett C, Feldman M, Richardson C: Reduction of 24-hour gastric acidity with combination drug therapy in patients with duodenal ulcer. Gastroenterology 77:1015, 1979
66. Walt RP, Male PJ, Rawlings J, et al: Comparison of the effects of Ranitidine, Cimetidine and placebo on the 24-hour gastric acidity and nocturnal acid secretion in patients with duodenal ulcer. Gut 22:49, 1981
67. Pounder RE, Williams JE, Hunt RH, et al: The effects of oral Cimetidine on food-stimulated gastric acid secretion and 24-hour intragastric acidity. *In* Cimetidine. Burland WL, Simkins MA, eds. pp 198–204. Amsterdam, Excerpta Medica, 1977
68. Galmiche JP, Vallot T, Mayeur S, et al: Effet de la Ranitidine sur le pH gastrique chez le sujet sain. Interet de l'en registrement continu sur 24 heures pour le choix du fractionnement optimal d'une dose therapeutique. Gastroenterol Clin Biol 6:352, 1982
69. McCarthy DM, Hyman PE: Testing antisecretory drugs in Zollinger-Ellison syndrome: Problems and limits in pharmacological studies. Dig Dis and Sci 27, 4:377, 1982
70. Vallot T, Mignon M, Mazure R, Bonfils S: Evaluation of antisecretory drug therapy of Zollinger-Ellison syndrome (ZES) using 24-hour pH monitoring. Dig Dis and Sci 28, 7:577, 1983
71. Malagelada JR: Uncertainties in the management of the Zollinger-Ellison syndrome. Gastroenterol 84:188, 1983
72. Richardson CT, Walsh JH: The value of a histamine $H_2$-receptor antagonist in the

management of patients with the Zollinger-Ellison syndrome. N Engl J Med 294:133, 1976

73. McCarthy DM, Hyman P: Effect of isopropamide on response to oral Cimetidine in patients with Zollinger-Ellison syndrome. Dig Dis and Sci 27:353, 1982

74. Mignon M, Vallot T, Calmiche JP, et al: Interest of a combined anti-secretory treatment, Cimetidine and Pirenzepine in the management of severe forms of Zollinger-Ellison syndrome. Digestion 20:56, 1981

75. Longdong W: Anticholinergics for peptic ulcer—a Renaissance. Hepatogastroenterology 29:40, 1982

76. Crane SA, Summers RW, Heeringa WG: Long-term Cimetidine and anticholinergic therapy in patients with gastrinoma. Am J Surgery 138:446, 1979

77. Allende HD, Bissonnette BM, Rafuman JP, et al: Progressive increase in drug requirement in the long-term management of patients with Zollinger-Ellison syndrome. Gastroenterol 82:1007, 1982

78. Freston JW: Drugs five years later: Cimetidine: II. Adverse reactions and patterns of use. Ann Int Med 97, 5:728, 1982

79. Mignon M, Vallot T, Hervoir P, et al: Ranitidine versus Cimetidine in the management of Zollinger-Ellison syndrome. *In* "Ranitidine," pp. 169–177. Proceedings of an International Symposium, World Congress of Gastroenterology, Stockholm, 1982, eds. Riley AJ and Salmon PR. Excerpta Medica, Amsterdam, 1982

80. Pedrazzoli S, Petrin P, Pasquali C, et al: Ranitidine reverses Cimetidine-induced mental confusion in a patient with Zollinger-Ellison syndrome. Arch Surg 118:256, 1983

81. Collen MJ, Howard JM, McArthur KE, et al: Comparison of Ranitidine and Cimetidine in the treatment of gastric hypersecretion. Ann Int Med 100:52, 1984

82. McCarthy DM: $H_2$-receptor antagonists in Zollinger-Ellison syndrome. Proceedings of International Symposium, "Update: $H_2$-Receptor Antagonists," London, 1983. Ed. Cohen S: Biomedical Information Corp, NY (in press, 6/84)

83. Raufman JP, Collen MJ, Howard JM, et al: Decreased parietal cell responsiveness to Cimetidine in some patients with ZES. Gastroenterol 84:1281A, 1983

84. Ziemniak JA, Madura M, Adamonis A, et al: Failure of Cimetidine in the Zollinger-Ellison syndrome. Dig Dis and Sci 28, 11:976, 1983

85. Rune SJ, Larsen NE, Stadil F, Worning H: Development of resistance to Cimetidine in a patient with Zollinger-Ellison syndrome. Gastroenterol 80:1265, 1981

86. Mignon M, Vallot T, Mayeur S, Bonfils S: Ranitidine and Cimetidine in Zollinger-Ellison syndrome. Brit J Clin Pharm 10:173, 1980

87. Bonfils S, Mignon M, Vallot T, Mayeur S: Use of Ranitidine in the medical treatment of Zollinger-Ellison syndrome. Scan J Gastro 16 (supp. 69):119, 1981

88. Mignon M, Vallot T, Bonfils S: Use of Ranitidine in the management of Zollinger-Ellison syndrome. *In* "The Clinical Use of Ranitidine," pp. 281–282. Proceedings of the Second International Symposium on Ranitidine, London, 1981, eds. Misiewiez JJ, Wormsley KG. The Medicine Publishing Found., Oxford, 1981

89. Lebert PA, McLeod SM, Mahon WA, et al: Ranitidine kinetics and dynamics: 1. Oral dose studies. Clin Pharm Ther 30:539, 1981

90. Hansen WE, Bertl S: Inhibition of cholinesterases by Ranitidine. Lancet (i):235, 1983

91. Scarpignato C, Bertaccini G: Different effects of Cimetidine and Ranitidine on gastric emptying in rats and man. Agents and Actions 12:1720, 1982

92. Danilewitz M, Tim LO, Hirschowitz B: Ranitidine suppression of gastric hypersecretion resistant to Cimetidine. N Engl J Med 306:20, 1982

93. Pearce P, Funder JW: Histamine $H_2$-receptor antagonists: Radioreceptor assay for antiandrogenic side effects. Clin Exp Pharmacol Physiol 7:442, 1980

94. Soll AH: An overall perspective—gastric acid secretion *in vivo* in histamine and gastric acid secretion. Smith, Klein and French International Co., Philadelphia, 1983

95. Lamers CB, Jansen JB: The effect of a gastrin receptor antagonist on gastric acid secretion and serum gastrin in the Zollinger-Ellison syndrome. J Clin Gastroent 5:21, 1983

96. Richardson CT, Feldman M, McClelland RN, et al: Effect of Vagotomy in Zollinger-Ellison syndrome. Gastroenterol 77:682, 1979

97. McCarthy DM, Peikin SR, Lopatin RN, et al: Hyperparathyroidism—a reversible cause of Cimetidine-resistant gastric hypersecretion. Brit Med J 1:1765, 1979

98. Basso N, Passaro E: Effect of calcium on pentagastrin, histamine, bethanecol and insulin-stimulated gastric secretion in the ferret. J Surg Res 13:32, 1972

99. Shimoda SS, Saunders DR, Rubin CE: The Zollinger-Ellison syndrome with steatorrhoea: The mechanism of fat and vitamin B12 malabsorption. Gastroenterol 55:705, 1968

100. Ippoliti AF, Isenberg JI, Hagie L: The effect of oral and intravenous 16,16-dimethyl prostaglandin $E_2$ in duodenal ulcer and Zollinger-Ellison syndrome patients. Gastroenterol 80:55, 1980

101. Hutton SW, Morley JE, Parent MK, et al: Thyrotropin-releasing hormone suppresses gastric acid output in patients with Zollinger-Ellison syndrome and systemic mastocytosis. Am J Med 71:957, 1981

102. Long RG, Barnes AJ, Adrian TE, et al: Suppression of pancreatic endocrine tumor secretion by long-acting somatostatin analogue. Lancet (2):764, 1979

103. Faller L, Jackson R, Malinowska D, et al: Mechanistic aspects of gastric $[H^+ + K^+]$-ATPase. *In* Transport ATPases, Annal NY Acad Sci 402:146, 1982

104. Lamers CBHW, Jansen JBMJ, Rune S, et al: Experience with omeprazole in the Zollinger-Ellison syndrome. Abstract *In* Proceedings of Symposium on Substituted Benzimidazoles. World Congress of Gastroenterology, Stockholm, June 1982

105. McArthur KE, Collen MJ, Cherner JA, et al: Omeprazole as a single daily dose is effective therapy in Zollinger-Ellison syndrome. Gastroenterol 86:1178, 1984 (in press)

106. Thompson JC, Lewis BG, Weiner I, Townsend CM: The role of surgery in the Zollinger-Ellison syndrome. Ann Surg 197:594, 1983

107. Stark DD, Moss AA, Goldberg HI, et al: Computed tomography and nuclear magnetic resonance imaging of pancreatic islet cell tumors. Surgery 94:1024, 1983

108. Freisen SR: Treatment of Zollinger-Ellison syndrome: A 25-year assessment. Am J Surg 143:331, 1982

109. Bonfils S, Mignon M, Gratton J: Cimetidine treatment of acute and chronic Zollinger-Ellison syndrome. World J Surg 3:587, 1979

110. Stage JG, Stadil F: The clinical diagnosis of Zollinger-Ellison syndrome. Scan J Gastroent 14 (supp. 53):79, 1979

111. Deveney CW, Deveney KS, Way LW: The Zollinger-Ellison syndrome—23 years later. Ann Surg 188:384, 1978

112. Barreras RF, Mack E, Goodfriend T, Damm M: Resection of gastrinoma in the Zollinger-Ellison syndrome. Gastroenterol 82:953, 1981

113. Bonfils S, Landor JH, Mignon M, Hervoir R: Results of surgical management of 92 consecutive patients with Zollinger-Ellison syndrome. Annal Surg 194(6):692, 1981

114. Friesen SR, Kimmel JR, Tomita T: Pancreatic polypeptide as a screening marker for pancreatic polypeptide tumors in multiple endocrinopathies. Am J Surg 139:61, 1980

115. Friesen SR: Tumors of the endocrine pancreas. N Engl J Med 306:58, 1982

116. Zollinger RM, Ellison C, Fabri PJ, et al: Primary peptic ulcerations of the jejunum associated with islet cell tumors. Ann Surg 192:422, 1980

117. Peters MN, Richardson CT, Feldman M, et al: Exploratory laparotomy, vagotomy and Cimetidine for treatment of Zollinger-Ellison syndrome (ZES). Gastroenterol 82:1149, 1982

118. McClelland R: Surgical approaches to Zollinger-Ellison syndrome. *In* Peptic Ulcer Disease—1983, American College of Gastroenterology, Manchester, MS

119. Richardson, CT, Peters, MN, Feldman, M, et al: Treatment of Zollinger–Ellison syndrome with proximal gastric vagotomy, exploratory laparotomy and $H_2$-receptor antagonists. Gastroenterol (in press)

# 3 | Glucagon-Producing Tumors

*Jens Juul Holst*

## INTRODUCTION

The case of glucagon-producing tumors provides a fine example of the impact of a suitable analytical tool on the incidence of a disease; although such tumors have been suspected since 1942,[1] there had been very few positive reports until Mallinson and co-workers in 1974 called attention to the association of a peculiar skin rash—the necrolytic migratory erythema—and glucagon-producing tumors.[2] The awareness of this skin rash as a cutaneous marker of internal malignancy and the availability in most countries of plasma analyses for glucagon opened the way for a large number of case reports, and it now seems that such tumors are as frequent as, for example, the tumors associated with the WDHA-syndrome (Chapter 6).

It is unlikely that the number of reports reflects a truly increased incidence, and this then tells us that a large number of cases must have passed unnoticed. It is not surprising that the skin rash has been falsely diagnosed (see below), but more so that the pancreatic tumors, which are often fairly large, have been overlooked. The explanation should probably be sought among the facts that many of the patients are elderly, that many have complications (pneumonia, thromboembolism) or exhibit gradual cachexia, which, in combination with pancreatic malignancy, does not raise suspicion of an *endocrine* tumor. Such considerations are probably still valid and would indicate that many cases still escape diagnosis. Thus, every effort to enhance the awareness of this often surgically curable condition is worthwhile.

This review will not attempt to present a complete record of cases published so far. Such compilations have appeared with regular intervals.[3-9] Their usefulness is limited by the fact that many, particularly early cases, are poorly documented and therefore unreliable, and by the fact that a large number of cases have been subject to double (or even triple) publication. The compilations may therefore be somewhat misleading. In this chapter emphasis is on general features of these tumors deduced from a critical study of the literature.

## MORPHOLOGY OF THE GLUCAGON-PRODUCING TUMORS

Precise classification of pancreatic endocrine cells was not possible until the advent of modern immunohistochemical methods, and older cases of alpha-2 cell tumors may therefore not be cases of glucagonomas. It follows that neither do older descriptions of such cases, in which other components of the glucagonoma syndrome are not mentioned, necessarily represent atypical cases. However, there is little doubt that glucagon-producing tumors may be found without an accompanying syndrome. In a very thorough study of 1366 adult autopsy cases Grimelius et al[10] found a tumor frequency of 0.8%, all of them adenomas, all of them containing histochemically defined glucagon cells. None of the adenomas had been suspected during life. Although it is not known whether or not these tumors were actually secreting glucagon, its probably fair to consider them early cases; this then tells us that a category of patients exists with glucagon-producing tumors, which probably show no symptoms (but in whom a diagnosis might be made with glucagon radioimmunoassay?). Glucagon-cell tumors or adenomas without an accompanying syndrome were also observed by Lomsky et al,[11] Warner et al,[12] and Bordi et al,[13] and Ruttman et al,[9] who concluded that glucagon-cell tumors from patients without the syndrome were benign, usually multiple, and with secretory granules (electron microscopy) that resemble normal islet A-cell granules. The tumors associated with the syndrome were typically large (3–35 cm), generally malignant, and frequently with atypical granule morphology (Fig. 3-1).[9,12-17]

The latter observation is important, because it tells us that a glucagon-producing tumor may not be classified correctly by electron microscopical characterization of granules, as is possible in normal islets (Fig. 3-1).[17] Although, hypothetically, in some tumors, peptide turnover could be so rapid that the peptide content of the tumor would be too low to allow immunohistochemical demonstration, there is little doubt that the best method for classification of the pancreatic endocrine tumors is immunohistochemistry, by which the secreted product is identified at the tissue level.[17,18]

The morphology of the larger glucagon-producing tumors show no outstanding features distinguishing them from other pancreatic endocrine tumors; typically they are pleomorphic with immunoreactive cells forming strands and ribbons.[7,8,17] Sometimes the tumors appear sclerotic and necrotic and in such cases the immunoreactive cells may be found compressed between large masses of connective tissue (Fig. 3-2).[19]

Most of the syndrome-associated tumors are malignant; although mitotic figures and nuclear atypia seem to be rare,[7,12,13] more than half of the tumors show

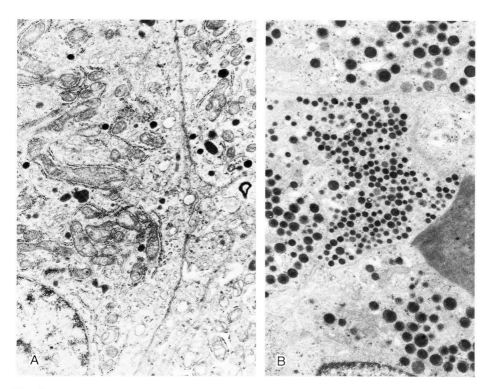

**Fig. 3-1.** Glucagonoma ultrastructure. (A) Electron micrograph of glucagonoma. Sections of three tumor cells are seen; the relatively few granules differ markedly from the granules of normal A-cells, shown in (B), which shows sections of three A-cells surrounding a $D_1$-cell. (A, B × 16,700). (By courtesy of Professor Lars-Inge Larsson, Institute of Pathology, University of Copenhagen, Denmark).

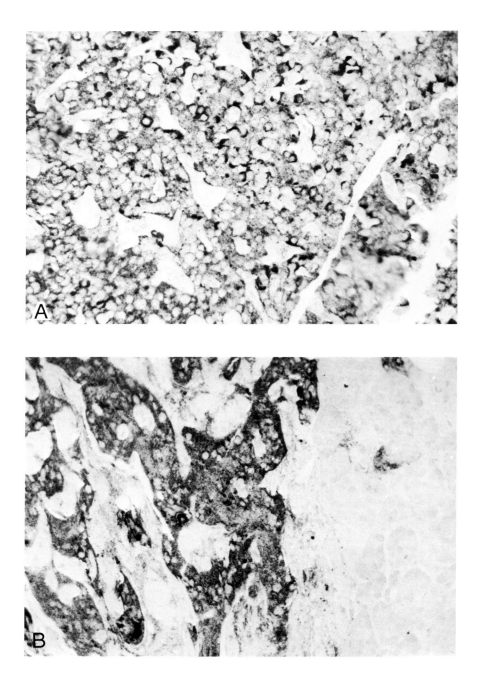

**Fig. 3-2.** Pancreatic glucagonomas. Immunoperoxidase studies. The figure shows the microscopical appearance of two glucagonomas, stained immunohistochemically with the peroxidase-antiperoxidase technique; material with glucagon-like immunoreactivity will appear dark with this technique.[17] (A) This tumor forms ribbons and strands consisting almost entirely of glucagon immunoreactive cells. (B) In this tumor, columns of tumor cells are seen compressed between exocrine or connective tissue. (A × 102, B × 69). (By courtesy of Professor Lars-Inge Larsson, Institute of Pathology, University of Copenhagen).

metastatic spread at the time of diagnosis,[7,8] typically to the liver and local lymph nodes. It is important to recall that multiple tumors may occur.[9-12]

## MIXED TUMORS

Typically the pancreatic endocrine tumors contain more than one peptide-producing cell type[17] and glucagonomas form no exception. The most common additional cell type seems to be the pancreatic polypeptide-producing cell,[12,13,20-22] but also insulin, [12,19,23,24] somatostatin,[13,19,25] and gastrin-producing cells may be found.[23,26-28] Likewise, glucagon cells may constitute part of tumors with predominant content of other cell types,[18,22,29,39] and glucagon-producing pancreatic adenomas may constitute part of multiple endocrine adenomatosis-type I,[9,13,31-34] some cases even presenting with a full glucagonoma syndrome.[23,35]

The important lesson of the latter observations is that other endocrine neoplasia must be sought for when the diagnosis of a glucagonoma is made. Not only must other glands than the pancreas be screened in the search for a MEA I syndrome, but also signs of multiple hormone production by the tumor itself are important to disclose, since metastatic spread may occur with cells which do not produce the original predominant peptide product. Thus, a typical insulinoma or gastrinoma case may be transformed into a glucagonoma syndrome after surgery,[27,29,36] and a successfully treated glucagonoma patient may later show the symptoms of an insulinoma.[37] Therefore, it is important that the tumor is correctly classified at the operation so that control determination of all tumor products can be arranged in the follow-up.

## EXTRAPANCREATIC TUMORS

There is an early observation by Unger and co-workers[38] on the presence of insulin and glucagon (in minute quantities) in bronchogenic metastases, but glucagon is usually not elevated in malignancies otherwise associated with ectopic hormone production (e.g., small cell lung carcinoma).[39] A duodenal glucagon-producing tumor in a patient presenting with what appeared to be a somewhat atypical syndrome was recently described.[40] There are two reports on kidney tumors which seem to have been producing glucagon-like substances.[41,42] One was later shown[43] to produce a peptide which resembled more the type of glucagon derived from the intestine (see ref. 44 for review). Intestinal type glucagon has been found with a high frequency in cells of human rectal carcinoids.[45,46] It is not known whether secretion from such tumors of "enteroglucagon" actually takes place or what the consequences of such secretion might be. The enteroglucagon-producing kidney tumor described above might have been responsible for the intestinal villous hypertrophy noted in the patient, who was admitted to the hospital because of marked intestinal stasis (and a transient erythematous skin rash!)[41] (see ref. 44 for recent review).

## AGE AND SEX

Although most cases have been described in middle-aged or elderly people, there are also descriptions of patients as young as 19 years.[47] Originally, it was felt that the typical glucagonoma patient was female, but the increasing number of observations allows the conclusion that both sexes are affected with equal frequency.[7,8]

## GENETICS

The multiple endocrine adenomatosis type I (MEA I, Wermers syndrome) is a familial disease, and if a glucagonoma is diagnosed in such a family, the other members of the family should have their plasma concentrations of glucagon measured. Indeed, such analysis may reveal more cases.[35] A familial hyperglucagonemia has also been described; one member had a classical glucagonoma syndrome, and elevated levels were found in 4 other members of the family without other symptoms.[48] The chromatographic glucagon profile in the non-affected members suggested that the elevation was due to high molecular weight material not necessarily related to glucagon biosynthesis (see below), and this "syndrome" therefore awaits further characterization.

We have had the opportunity to follow for 7 years the homozygotic twin of one of our typical glucagonoma syndrome patients; at no time has she had any symptoms of a glucagonoma nor elevation of plasma glucagon.[49]

## THE GLUCAGONOMA SYNDROME

The exact role of glucagon in the control of metabolism has been a matter of some controversy over the years, and this undoubtedly explains why it was quite difficult to predict the disturbances caused by excessive secretion of that hormone. Indeed, it was surprising to learn that the most conspicuous component of the glucagonoma syndrome was a skin rash![2] But the element of surprise was probably only due to our ignorance of the physiology of glucagon, as will be evident. The most important components of the syndrome are listed in Table 3-1 and will be described in detail below.

**Table 3-1.** Typical Features of the Glucagonoma Syndrome

Glucagon-producing tumor of the pancreas
Skin rash: migratory necrolytic erythema (including stomatitis, sore tongue, cheilitis, vaginitis and nail changes)
Panhypo-aminoacidemia
Variable glucose intolerance
Renal glucosuria
Anemia
Weight loss
Hypersedimentation
Thromboembolism
Psychiatric disturbances

## The Skin Rash: Migratory Necrolytic Erythema

The first description of what is today known as the glucagonoma syndrome was given in 1942 by Becker, Kahn and Rothman, who gave a detailed description of the clinical course and the skin rash, and noted that the patient also had an islet cell type of pancreatic carcinoma.[1] Actually, their case is very typical for the syndrome, but the authors were in no position to associate the clinical condition with hyperproduction of glucagon. Neither was this possible for MacGavran and co-workers when they published the first proven case of a glucagon-producing tumor—proven because of their use of the recently developed radioimmunoassay for glucagon to demonstrate hyperglucagonemia and a high glucagon content of the tumor.[50] These authors noted in their patient a "chronic eczematoid or bullous dermatitis," but they felt that it might be an incidental part of the syndrome and did not compare the dermatitis (said to defy specific diagnosis) to earlier descriptions of similar cases (see 3 or 7 for references). Thus, it fell to the lot of a group of British dermatologists and gastroenterologists to disclose the association between glucagon hypersecretion and the very peculiar skin rash, named necrolytic migratory erythema after Wilkinson.[2,51-54] Excellent descriptions of the skin rash

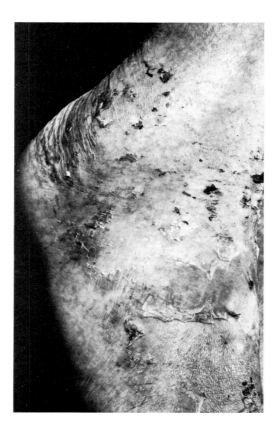

**Fig. 3-3.** Necrolytic migratory erythema. The figure shows crust and hyperpigmentations and a ruptured bulla. (By courtesy of Dr. N. Bang Pedersen, Lasarettet i Lund).

have been presented by Wilkinson[51] and Sweet.[52] Detailed discussions of the subject have been given.[7,37,55] Macroscopically, the skin lesion starts as annular or figurate erythema at intertriginous and periorificial sites. The erythema becomes raised, and the central parts form superficial bullae. The roofs of the bullae detach, leaving exuding erosive areas encircled by serous crusts (Fig. 3-3). The lesions become confluent and thus serpiginious (Fig. 3-4). The face, the trunk, and, in particular, areas exposed to traumas may also be involved. The lesions heal within two or three weeks, typically leaving hyperpigmentation. The lesion thus reminds one of superficial burns. The eruption is chronic and recurrent with spontaneous remissions and exacerbations. Thus, at different sites lesions may be found in different stages, often confusing the picture. Perioral and paranasal crusting, often with extension onto forehead and cheeks, is frequently present. Angular cheilitis is a very common feature and so is nail dystrophy. Almost all patients have had a painful red glossitis, which may be very troublesome; the sore tongue may well be the cause of their first visit to the doctor. Inflammatory vulvovaginitis may also be seen. Scrapings

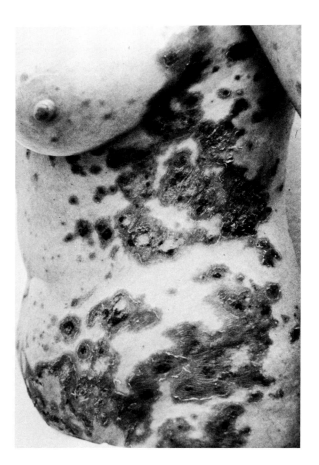

**Fig. 3-4.** Necrolytic migratory erythema. The figure shows the gyrate and serpignious configurations which upon confluence of the lesions. Also note hyperpigmentation and crusting. (Helland S, Thorsen E, Holst JJ, Ingemansson S: Glukagonomsyndromet- nekrolytisk migrerende erythem. Tidsskr Nor Lægeforen 99: 638, 1979)

and cultures of the involved mucous membranes frequently reveal secondary infection with Candida.[37,47,56]

## Histology

Some authors believe that histopathologically the lesions show merely nonspecific spongiotic dermatitis. However, in early lesions, at least if superinfection has not occurred, a rather typical picture is seen,[51,52,53,55,57] particularly if the

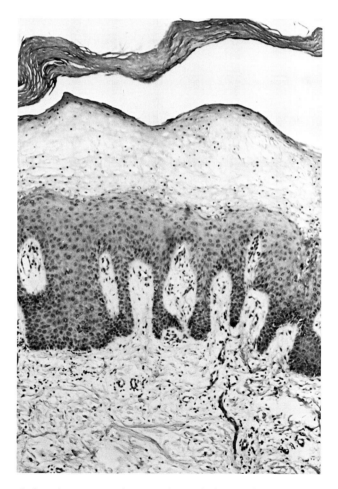

**Fig. 3-5.** Necrolytic migratory erythema. Histopathology. There is a marked spongiosis and necrosis in the upper layers of the stratum malphigi, separating a thin parakeratotic layer below the pre-existing stratum corneum and the acanthotic lower layers of the epidermis. (Pedersen NB, Jonsson L, Holst JJ: Necrolytic migratory erythema and glucagon cell tumour of the pancreas: the glucagonoma syndrome. Acta Dermatovener (Stockholm) 56:391, 1976)

biopsy is taken from the edge of a lesion. A typical lesion is shown in Figure 3-5. It shows the marked superficial spongiosis and necrosis, leading to cleft formations. The granular layer is lost and there is a thin parakeratotic layer below the pre-existing stratum corneum. There is an impression of "sudden death" of the cells of the upper layer of the stratum Malphigi. Note the pyknosis of the ballooning cells. Typical also is the acanthosis and the perivascular leukocyte infiltration of the dermis. Acantholysis is notably absent. Thus the lesion is essentially epidermal with subcorneal blister formation.

## Hypoaminoacidemia

Already Mallinson and co-workders[2] noted that in all of 4 patients, in whom this was investigated, the levels of plasma amino acids were strikingly low, and in fact they suggested this as a pathogenetic mechanism for the skin rash. A large number of later reports have confirmed this observation.[4,5,7,15,16,24,35,55,58-71] As already noted by Mallinson et al,[2] the levels may vary with the intensity of the disease, but the hypoaminoacidemia is so constant a finding and so pronounced that it may be diagnostic. Usually, all individual amino acids are subnormal, but there are reports that glutamic acid and isoleucine levels may be normal.[24,64,65]

The hypo-aminoacidemia is probably a consequence of excessive glucagon secretion.[80] One of the most remarkable effects of glucagon, even in physiological concentrations, is to decrease plasma levels of amino acids.[72-75] Usually, glucagon's effect is most pronounced on the levels of the glycogenic amino acids, whereas branched-chain amino acids are less affected; there is some uncertainty about this, however.[74,76] Possibly, a chronic, maintained hypo-aminoacidemia eventually causes depression of other amino acids as well. In addition, the effect in glucagonoma patients on branched-chain amino acids may be second to an effect of hyperglucagonemia on glucose and insulin turnover.[75]

The hypo-aminoacidemia is alleviated if the glucagon-producing-tumor is successfully removed by surgery.[24,61,65,66,69] or upon successful chemotherapy.[61,69] Furthermore, pancreatectomy in man, believed to decrease the plasma levels of glucagon, leads to increased concentrations of exactly those amino acids that are most sensible to the concentration-lowering effects of glucagon.[77-79]

The hypo-aminoacidemia has been associated with the pathogenesis of the skin rash, and indeed there is good reason to believe that the low levels of amino acids are responsible. Protein malnutrition is known to cause in some instances a similar skin rash,[81-83] but the strongest argument for the relationship comes from the excellent effect on the skin rash of restoration of the plasma amino acid concentrations by parenteral nutrition.[63,70] During such treatment, glucagon concentrations, if anything, went up, proving that the skin rash was not an effect of glucagon itself. In a single report,[84] the skin rash improved repeatedly after 7–10 days treatment with a 5% dextrose in halfnormal saline infusion (and insulin); amino acid levels were not reported. It is known, however, that carbohydrates influence amino acid utilization in man, and the effect of the dextrose in this report may have been due to an increased amino acid availability.[85] In a single report[86] a skin rash appeared after glucagon treatment of what was believed to be a case of acute pancreatitis; neither skin histology nor amino acid levels were reported, however.

## Glucose Intolerance

Because of glucagon's notorious effect on glucose metabolism, a diabetogenic effect of glucagonomas has been looked for since the first proven case in the literature,[50] and indeed most authors have included diabetes among the key components of the syndrome. Nevertheless, diabetes or just glucose intolerance is a much less constant feature of the syndrome than is the hypo-aminoacidemia.[65] Considering the effects of experimental hyperglucagonemia on glucose metabolism, this would also be the expected outcome. Studies of the effects of glucagon infusion in normal subjects (subjects who can respond with increased insulin secretion) have shown that the hyperglycemic effect of the infusion is transient,[87] and that glucose tolerance is not affected by such infusion.[88] In other words, glucagon's dramatic effect on glucose metabolism depends (partly) on the prevailing insulin concentrations. Major disturbances in glucose metabolism in glucagonoma patients would therefore not be expected. Indeed, a number of observations support this view.

First of all, far from all glucagonoma patients have diabetes mellitus or even glucose intolerance.[6,7] Quite a number have had completely normal blood glucose values in spite of greatly increased glucagon levels.[2,4,16,37,47,58,60,65,89,90] Secondly, various treatments of the patients, which have resulted in definite changes in glucagon levels, have not brought about "expected" changes in glucose metabolism: (1) In some cases, glucose intolerance has persisted after surgical removal of the tumor or other successful treatment with normalization of glucagon levels.[15,62,65,66,91,92] (2) In some cases glucose tolerance was even impaired after such treatment.[24,65] (3) In some cases the diabetes could very well be explained by insulin deficiency.[15,93,94] On the whole, it is difficult to disregard the possibility that (a) a sometimes very large islet cell carcinoma of the pancreas might bring about diabetes like other pancreatic adenocarcinomas or (b) that either extensive surgery on the pancreas (frequent treatment of glucagonomas) or treatment with the beta-cell poison streptozotocin might cause insulinopenia with subsequent diabetes. Indeed, the reported cases of ketoacidosis in glucagonoma patients[84,93,94] are probably best explained this way. (4) Finally, there is no correlation between the degree of diabetes and glucagon levels of the patients.[6]

Kahn et al. infused a somatostatin-analog which markedly depressed glucagon levels in a glucagonoma patient; this, however, had no effect on blood glucose.[95] A more direct approach was adopted by Boden, Wilson and Owen, who examined net splanchnic glucose and ketone body production in a glucagonoma patient by catheterization technique before and after complete tumor resection.[96] Whereas the hyperglucagonemia could be held responsible for an increase in ketone body production, it was impossible to demonstrate any effect on splanchnic glucose production (although it was possible that glucagon was responsible for a larger fractional contribution of gluconeogenesis before operation). In a similar study, Nankervis et al. studied glucose kinetics using $^3$H-3-glucose infusions in a glucagonoma patient before and after complete resection.[97] Glucose kinetics were unchanged, and glucose tolerance was unaffected by hyperglucagonemia.[97]

Condon[98] reported long-term high-dose glucagon treatment of patients with Paget's disease, and noted that none of the patients developed glucose intolerance as a consequence of the treatment. Part of the explanation of the inconspicuous effect may be so-called down-regulation, desensitization, elicited by the very large concentrations of glucagon in these patients.[99] Thus, Nankervis et al observed that a glucagon infusion which, after removal of the tumor, elicited a marked cAMP response was ineffective before operation.[97] Similarly, intravenous injection of 1 mg of glucagon (a very large dose) did not bring about a hyperglycemic response in some of these patients.[50,92,100] In other studies, 1 mg of glucagon elicited a normal glucose response, but this was felt to be due to the extremely large concentrations of glucagon resulting from such injection.[23,65] Apparently, very high concentrations may break the desensitization in some cases.

It remains to be explained why the removal of the glucagon-producing tumors have improved glucose tolerance in some cases.[2,4,5,56,61,65,101,102] In all of these, the patients were obviously diabetic preoperatively, and the most natural explanation would be that, at the same time, they suffered from absolute or relative insulin deficiency. Very few studies have considered this possibility, which therefore is difficult to evaluate from the literature reports. However, it is well established that the liver is extremely sensitive to glucagon in insulin deficiency,[88] and in such cases it is probable that glucagon excess may have contributed to glucose intolerance.

As discussed above, many of the glucagonomas are mixed tumors, and some of them contain and secret somatostatin. Somatostatin, which appears to have little activity on liver metabolism, is likely to inhibit insulin secretion and might be another cause of a relative insulin deficiency in such cases. On the other hand, some of the glucagonomas probably secret insulin also, and in such cases a deterioration of glucose tolerance would be expected to occur after removal of the tumor.[23,24,65]

Thus glucose intolerance is not an invariant part of the glucagonoma syndrome, and if present, actually should call for further investigations to unveil the underlying causes.

## Renal Glycosuria

A number of investigators have observed marked renal glycosuria in glucagonoma patients.[2,16,47,89,101] This seems to occur early and might be a direct effect of glucagon on the kidneys. This finding, therefore, deserves further investigation. Obviously, renal glycosuria in these patients should not be taken as an indication of hyperglycemia or diabetes.

## Other Features

Apart from the tumor, the skin rash, the hypoaminoacidemia, and the disturbances of glucose metabolism, there are a number of other features that are less specific, and maybe less easily associated with glucagon excess, but which are sufficiently serious and frequent to warrant attention.

*Weight Loss.*  This is very constant finding and may be profound. The weight loss is prominent also in cases with smaller tumors without mestastatic spread,[2,4,5,49,61,62,64,69] suggesting that the cachexia is a consequence of the catabolic actions of glucagon excess, and not merely tumor-associated. In support of this, glucagon in high concentrations has been found to increase ureagenesis partly at the expense of the free amino acid pool and partly by hydrolysis of visceral protein,[73,74,76] but it is not known if other mechanisms are also operative.

*Anemia.*  The anemia, which is usually normochromic and normocytic, is also a constant finding, and frequently severe, requiring transfusion therapy. When investigated, serum iron, serum B12, and folate have been normal, and the anemia has not responded to therapy with any of these moieties. The anemia also responds to successful tumor therapy.[58,60,103] Again, anemia may be a direct effect of glucagon excess. Prolonged therapy with long-acting glucagon (protamine zinc) markedly depressed erythropoiesis in rats and mice.[104] It was suggested that glucagon was acting at the level of erythroid stem cell differentiation. Surprisingly low concentrations were active, considerably lower than those found in most glucagonoma patients,[104] suggesting that anemia found in other clinical conditions with hyperglucagonemia (renal failure, liver cirrhosis, chronic inflammation) might also be associated with glucagon excess.

*Thromboembolism.*  Deep venous trombosis and pulmonary emboli occur in a very substantial number of patients, and in a conspicuous number of cases has been the cause of death.[1,2,12,15,16,29,35,40,49,51,57,71,89,102,105] This complication occurs without any other signs of coagulation defects and is not seen with the other endocrine tumors of the pancreas. Glucagon is not known to influence coagulation, but this has not been subjected to systematic study. This complication, which may be fatal, represents one of the main indications for active therapy and should be taken into consideration even if it is felt that the other features of the syndrome are tolerated reasonably well.

*Psychiatric Disturbances.*  Several authors have recorded psychiatric problems in their glucagonoma patients.[1,2,47,57,64,90,100,106] The disturbances have been mentioned very briefly, and thus defy classification; most of the cases have been dominated by depression. Whether this is a specific effect of glucagon excess is not known; some cases probably are well explained on the basis of the chronic debilitating condition and the skin rash that is probably being felt as socially inacceptable.

Neurological complications have been noted in some cases. Khandekar et al. (1939) reported the presence of optic atrophy, nystagmus, ataxia, and mild dysarthria in a glucagonoma patient, in whom larger, space-filling intracerebral processes were excluded. The neurological impairment was much improved after successful chemotherapy. One of the patients presented by Prinz et al.[69] was admitted to hospital for a bilateral scotoma, which regressed completely after successful surgery for a glucagonoma, and Lefebvre et al.[93] described in their patient neuropathy of the lower extremities, which improved after therapy.

*Other Symptoms.*  A number of patients have been complaining about epigastric fulness, gastric pain, and loss of appetite. Considering the size of the glucagonomas, which in some cases may fill a large part of the upper abdominal cavity, this is not surprising. Diarrhea[2,4,51,55,60,69,70,94,95,100] and vomiting[35,51,64,84] have been reported in some cases, but does not seem to be the rule, since in many cases

**Table 3-2.** Differential Diagnosis of the Skin Rash of the Glucagonoma Syndrome*

Pemphigus foliaceus
Asteatotic eczema
Autoeczematization
Toxic epidermal necrolysis
Subcorneal pustular dermatosis (Sneddon-Wilkinson)
Generalized pustular psoriasis
Acrodermatitis enteropathica
Mucocutaneous candidiasis
Chronic erythema multiforme
Nonspecific dermatitis
Pemphigoid
Chronic benign familial pemphigus (Hailey-Hailey disease)
Dermatophyte infections
Dermatitis herpetiformis
Erosive psoriasiform dermatitis
Seborrhoic dermatitis
Erythema annulare centrifugum
Herpes
Chemical burns (self-inflicted)
Pellagra

* This list also includes suggestions made prior to the establishment of the glucagonoma syndrome diagnosis.

this has explicitly not been found. In a number of cases severe exocrine pancreatic dysfunction (2) was seen, probably a mechanical consequence of tumor, which may help to explain the diarrhoea.

**Diagnosis.** The typical debut has been the sudden appearance of a skin rash. In retrospect, however, a number of patients were admitted for elucidation of glucosuria or glucose intolerance. The latter symptoms are sufficiently unspecific not to raise anybody's suspicion of a glucagon-producing tumor, and a screening for hyperglucagonemia at this stage is unrealistic. The typical skin rash will therefore in most cases be the first clue to the diagnosis. However, the literature reports show that most patients suffer for several years before the correct diagnosis is made. The list of diagnoses made on skin lesions, later shown to be the necrolytic migratory erythema of the glucagonoma syndrome is impressively long (Table 3-2) and includes almost every group of skin diseases. One of the greatest problems is superinfection, which seems to occur now and then (but not always) in most cases. Candida infections are particularly common.[37,47,56] Many cases also show periodical infections with *Staphylococcus aureus*,[37,47,57] in which cases pustules may dominate the picture.

The most closely resembling lesion is probably pemphigus foliaceus, which may have exactly the same macroscopical appearance. However, there is typically no acantholysis in the glucagonomas syndrome, and positive immunofluorescense should identify the pemphigus.[107] Chronic benign familial pemphigus may be suspected but should also be distinguishable by its extensive acantholysis. Another very similar condition is found in acrodermatitis enteropathica, today known to be caused by zinc deficiency.[108-110] However, in the glucagonoma patients there are usually normal serum zinc levels, and zinc therapy has no effect on the disease.[4,65]

Rockl et al.[37] discussed the so-called staphylodermia superficialis circinata and felt that the necrolytic migratory erythema belongs to this group of "cutaneous paraneoplasias," which were regarded as consequences of superficial staphylococcal skin infection in patients with impaired resistance because of internal malignancy. As discussed above, in many cases the necrolytic migratory erythema has appeared sterile, and it seems that the hypoaminoacidemia is the most natural pathogenic mechanism. Another bullous lesion of the epidermis, the pathogenesis of which is associated with microbial infection, is toxic epidermal necrolysis,[111] which will probably be distinguished from the glucagonoma syndrome by the age of the patients and the acute character of the disease.

Since diabetes is one of the entries to the diagnosis of the glucagonoma syndrome it is of interest to consider also the so-called bullosis diabeticorum.[112-114] This condition reportedly does not show the migratory behavior of the glucagonoma rash, but apart from that is sufficiently similar to warrant a plasma glucagon analysis to be carried out.

## Pseudoglucagonoma Syndrome

A number of reports of what appear to be typical necrolytic migratory erythema cases without a simultaneously occurring glucagonoma have now been described.[36,115,116] In one such case[116] there was also hyperglucagonemia due to cirrhosis of the liver and/or staphyloccous infection. Also, in this patient plasma levels of amino acids were low. Goodenberger's two patients both suffered from enteropathy, and one had generally low levels of plasma amino acids, which might explain the skin rash, but both had normal glucagon levels. Similar cases (but without plasma glucagon determinations) were presented by Thivolet et al.[117] and Rockl et al.[37]

## Glucagon Determination

Once suspected, the diagnosis of a glucagon-producing tumor is established by determination of the glucagon concentration in plasma. Glucagon radioimmunoassays are being performed in most countries today, and most research laboratories willingly assay such samples.

As discussed above, glucagon determination should be made in all cases where a chronic bullous skin rash has defied other diagnosis, or is resistant to rational therapy. The concentration of glucagon in plasma from glucagonoma patients is usually extremely elevated, and the suspected diagnosis is thus easily confirmed. Glucagon concentrations in glucagonoma cases and in other clinical conditions were compared by Leichter.[6] The mean value in 23 cases of proven glucagonomas was 2110 +/334 pg/ml ($\pm$ SEM), well above any other clinical conditions (the condition with the second highest concentration of glucagon was bacteremia or septicemia with 409 +/− 29 pg/ml). In our hands (13 Scandinavian cases) there has been no overlap whatsoever with the ranges of glucagon observed in any other condition, including cirrhosis of the liver. Conceivably, however, cases may be found in which the plasma concentration is not decisive. In such cases the finding by Stacpoole et al.[35] that secretin elicited what was considered a paradoxical increase in glucagon might be of interest as a clinically useful test. Unfortunately, the secretin preparation used was impure (Boots), the dose very large (2 U/kg), and control experiments were not performed. Thus, further evaluation of the test will be necessary.

## Heterogeneity

Much interest has been attached to the chromatographic profile of plasma glucagon in glucagonoma patients, because it was felt that elevations of the so-called proglucagon component might be of diagnostic value as in cases of insulin-producing tumors.[118,119] Indeed, it seems that there are elevated concentrations of a component in plasma which is larger than the true hormone of 3485 MW in many of the patients.[16,24,35,59,91,106,120-123] However, as shown recently, the pattern may differ considerably among patients (Fig. 3-6),[121] and in some the "proglucagon" component may not be elevated at all.

It is of greater interest to know if some patients escape diagnosis because of incomplete processing of the glucagon precursor. Today, in all laboratories, pancreatic glucagon is being determined by region-specific radioimmunoassays directed against the C-terminus of the molecule (to avoid interference by gut-derived glucagon). Since the glucagon precursor is extended at the C-terminal end of the glucagon sequence, it will not be measurable with such assays.[44] Thus there might exist tumors with incomplete processing at the C-terminus in which case the hyperglucagonemia will be immeasurable with the usual assays.[124] It might therefore be advisable to perform simultaneously an assay for the midregion of glucagon, which will measure all precursor forms.[44] Indeed, most plasma samples from these patients will show higher concentrations when measured in the latter assay system, indicating that such incomplete processing exists (Fig. 3-6).[121]

There is a single report[48] about a family with elevated concentrations of a very high-molecular-weight form of glucagon and no elevations of the other components (except in one single member, who was eventually shown to harbor a glucagonoma). Recent progress in the study of glucagon biosynthesis[125] has confirmed that the large glucagon precursor would have a molecular size considerably less than the former. The high-molecular-weight component is therefore difficult to relate to glucagon biosynthesis at present. In this discussion it might be useful to point out that the value of proinsulin determination in the diagnosis of an insulinoma lies in cases with near normal insulin concentrations; in such cases elevated concentrations of proinsulin may help to diagnose correctly the patient's hypoglycemic attacks. But turning to glucagonomas, we know of no cases with normal concentrations of glucagon in plasma; it may be that in the future the pancreatic adenomas discussed above, which are not associated with the other components of the syndrome, could be revealed with the aid of profile analysis. However, it may be questioned whether such patients were not better off without any diagnosis at all (note also that patients with necrolytic migratory erythema and normal plasma concentrations of glucagon so far have not been shown to harbor a glucagon-producing tumor!).

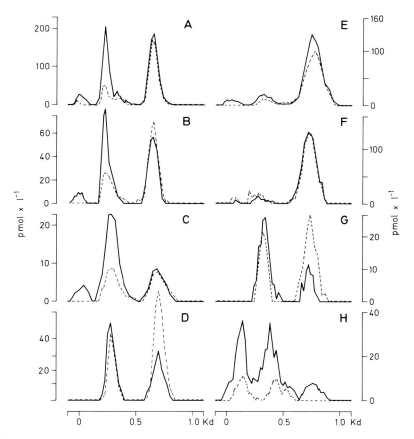

**Fig. 3-6.** Gel filtration profile on immunoreactive glucagon in plasma samples from 8 patients with glucagonoma syndrome. Gel filtrations were carried out on Sephadex G 50, and glucagon immunoreactivity was determined with region specific radioimmunoassays against the C-terminal sequence ($\cdots\cdots\cdots$) and the mid-sequence (———) of the glucagon molecule. Note that the two assays will measure different forms and different quantities of glucagon immunoreactivity; note also the heterogeneity of the profiles. (Holst JJ: Molecular heterogeneity of glucagon in normal subjects and in patients with glucagon-producing tumors. Diabetologia 24:359, 1983)

## Bioactivity

One suggested explanation of the modest effect of the hyperglucagonemia has been that the product of some glucagonomas might have decreased biological activity. However, several studies have indicated that at least the component corresponding in size with glucagon has also full bioactivity.[24,89,91,121] The "proglucagon" component was reported to have decreased activity (22%)[91] and did not interact with liver cell glucagon receptors,[121] but these findings cannot explain the inconspicuous effect of hyperglucagonemia, since in most cases the glucagon-sized component is predominating.[121]

## Functional Tests

A number of functional tests derived from studies of normal glucagon cell function have been employed in the study of glucagonoma patients, obviously with the purpose of disclosing peculiarities about secretion, which might be of diagnostic value; as already discussed, there really is no need for such tests at present. Furthermore, the results have been variable. Arginine infusions may[16,23,24,35,65,91,92,95,100,126] or may not[65] stimulate glucagon secretion (it is more interesting when ineffective!). Glucose may increase,[23,24,69,97] decrease,[65,91,94] or have no effect on glucagon concentrations.[60,65,95,100,126] Insulin infusions have had little effect or even a depressing effect, which is interesting.[16,23,95,100] Somatostatin inhibits glucagon secretion just as in normals.[23,35,65,95] Tolbutamide stimulates glucagon secretion,[24,92,100,126] but it is uncertain whether this is abnormal. Thus, although a few cases have demonstrated paradoxical responses to standard stimuli this is not the rule, and from a diagnostic point of view, these tests have been of little help.[65]

A high erythrocyte sedimentation rate is a regular finding; in fact there is not a single case with normal or mildly elevated levels. Thus a normal rate probably excludes the diagnosis of a glucagonoma.

## Tumor Localization

In some cases the tumors have been sufficiently large to allow localization by abdominal palpation, but in most cases the usual methods of localization of pancreatic tumors will be called for. However, as discussed above most of the tumors are rather large and would not escape palpation of the pancreas in the hands of a trained surgeon[127] and indeed no reported tumor has. It seems that laparotomy is also the only safe method of evaluation of possible spread. And finally, operative debulking of the tumor tissue has been beneficial, so that an operation seems to be indicated in all cases.

Nevertheless, there are many efficient ways of localizing these tumors (Fig. 3-7). The standard procedure would be selective angiography which (particularly on postoperative revision of films) will reveal most tumors.[128,129] However, a number of tumors have escaped detection with this technique,[19,70] and also ultrasound and computerized axial tomography has proven ineffective in some cases.[6,19,70,130,131]

In such cases one may turn to pancreatic vein catherization with phlebography and blood sampling for glucagon determination.[19,132] In many cases it is possible to localize with great precision the site of glucagon hyperproduction (Fig. 3-8). In addition, this examination may give some indication as to the presence and localization of glucagon-secreting metastatic deposits. For the surgeon it may be helpful to learn the particular pancreatic vein anatomy of that patients before enucleation of the tumor if this is possible.[19,132]

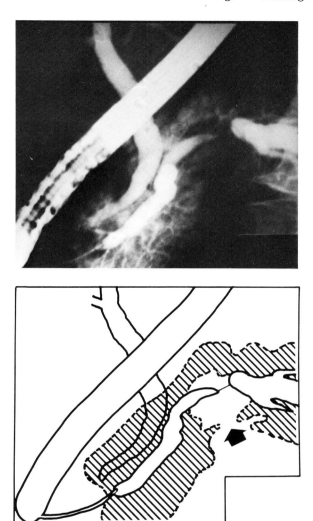

**Fig. 3-7.** Localization of glucagon-producing tumor. Result of endoscopic retrograde cholangio-pancreatography. The tumor which is situated in the corpus of the pancreas compresses the pancreatic duct to a thin thread; there is a marked prestenotic dilatation of the duct. (By courtesy of Dr. Peter Matzen, Hvidovre Hospital, Denmark).

## Treatment

Although probably all glucagon-producing tumors have the potential of giving off metastases, they are very slowly growing; documentation exists that patients have been doing reasonably well for more than ten years with the tumor and no treatment.[133] Therefore, the presence of metastases should not make the therapeutist give up.

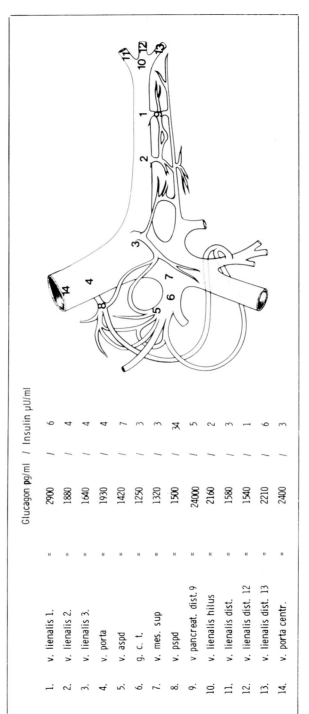

|   |   | Glucagon pg/ml | / | Insulin μU/ml |
|---|---|---|---|---|
| 1. | v. lienalis 1. | = | 2900 / | 6 |
| 2. | v. lienalis 2. | = | 1880 / | 4 |
| 3. | v. lienalis 3. | = | 1640 / | 4 |
| 4. | v. porta | = | 1930 / | 4 |
| 5. | v. aspd | = | 1420 / | 7 |
| 6. | g. c. t. | = | 1250 / | 3 |
| 7. | v. mes. sup | = | 1320 / | 3 |
| 8. | v. pspd | = | 1500 / | 34 |
| 9. | v. pancreat. dist. 9 | = | 24000 / | 5 |
| 10. | v. lienalis hilus | = | 2160 / | 2 |
| 11. | v. lienalis dist. | = | 1580 / | 3 |
| 12. | v. lienalis dist. 12 | = | 1540 / | 1 |
| 13. | v. lienalis dist. 13 | = | 2210 / | 6 |
| 14. | v. porta centr. | = | 2400 / | 3 |

**Fig. 3-8.** Localization of glucagon-producing tumor. Result of pancreatic phebography and selective catherization of pancreatic veins with sampling of blood for glucagon analysis. A striking arteriovenous gradient was found at position 9, one of the distal pancreatic veins. At the operation a 3 × 4 × 5 cm tumor was found in the tail of the pancreas and a hemipancreatectomy was performed. (Ingemansson S, Holst J, Larsson LI, Lunderquist A: Localization of glucagonomas by catheterization of the pancreatic veins and with glucagon assay. Surg Gynecol Obstet 145:504, 1977)

Approximately 50% of the patients have metastases at the time of diagnosis; this must be taken into account upon the planning of treatment. Surgical reval of the tumor has been performed successfully in a large number of cases[4,5,16,19,24,49,55,56,57,59,61,62,64,71,93,97,101,106] and at least a couple of years may pass without any signs of recurrence. However, a number of patients show recurrence in spite of what seemed initially a complete removal of the primary tumor and absence of deposits.[15,47,55,59,69,93,102] Also, 4 and 5 years after the removal of the tumor, two of our patients[49,57] have shown increasing concentrations of glucagon in plasma indicating (slow) recurrence. Hopefully, some of the operated patients will remain cured (a report of successful 12 years survival exist[5]), but it seems that the original optimism as to the success of operative removal was somewhat premature. However, there is no doubt that, if at all feasible, operation should be performed; not only may the operation delay the development of debilitating stages[133] but surgical debulking may have beneficial effects.[35,67,102,122]

Fortunately, a number of studies on the effect of various chemotherapeutic agents have been encouraging. The first drug to be tried was streptozotocin, a nitrosourea-based compound that is isolated from streptomyces achromogenes. The drug is only slightly active against the common human tumors, but was shown in 1968 to be active in the treatment of a patient with a mixed islet cell carcinoma[134]; eventually, that tumor also produced glucagon. Further studies in islet cell tumors were encouraging.[135] Streptozotocin has been reported to be effective in glucagonomas also, when used in doses varying from 0.5 to 1.5 $g/m^2 \times$ week.[58,91,102] However, later evaluation of the same patients, and a number of recent attempts, have been very disappointing.[15,26,55,60,70,84,96,136] There is a single report on the combination of streptozotocin with 5-fluorouracil, a combination which was very effective in the treatment of a gastrinoma syndrome[137]; in the glucagonoma case there was complete remission of the tumor and lasting normalization of plasma glucagon on a combination of 0.4 g $/m^2$ streptozotocin and 5-fluorouracil 0.45 $g/m^2$ for 4 days given in five series separated by 5 weeks.[103]

More success has been obtained with the use of dimethyl triazeno imidazole carboxamide (DTIC), which was first used by Kessinger, Lemon, and Foley,[60] after unsuccessful attempts to control a metastatic glucagonoma with streptozotocin. The dose was 250 $mg/m^2$ i.v. daily for 5 days every 4 weeks. There was an immediate improvement of the rash and near normalization of glucagon levels.

The reported follow-up period was 2 years. Similarly fine results were reported in more patients.[69,84,136] One of these was previously treated with a combination of cyclophosphamid, vincristine, and prednisone without success. However, there have also been less successful attempts; Stacpoole et al.[35] had to abstain from further DTIC treatment because of severe thrombopenia, and in the patients described by Hallengren et al.[70] and Duncan et al.[138] with severe metastatic tumors, DTIC was ineffective.

In all of the successful cases of DTIC-treatment, this has been preceded by other chemotherapeutic treatments, and it cannot be excluded that it is the combination of drugs which has caused the success, but otherwise there is little doubt that DTIC is the drug of choice at present. Probably, it would be advisable to institute such treatment also in cases where an apparently complete removal of tumor has been carried out; at least, chemotherapy is recommended if plasma glucagon is not completely normalized.

Embolization of coeliac artery branches to a metastatic glucagonoma has also been attempted.[28]

## Follow Up

The single most important thing to do is to determine the concentration of glucagon in plasma with regular intervals. Recurrences will invariably show early elevations. In this case a renewed evaluation of the case is called for, and it might be helpful to employ liver vein catheterizations and transhepatic percutaneous angiography with blood sampling and glucagon analysis in an attempt to localize the site of glucagon production.[19] Probably, however, chemotherapy will then be indicated rather than surgery.

In cases where treatment for some reason is unsuccessful, symptomatic treatment of the patients is necessary. As discussed above, there may be excellent effect of treatment designed to restore normal concentrations of amino acids in plasma.[63] In a recent case we have had reasonable success in treating a patient with a combination of bimonthly infusions of mixtures of amino acids, and, in between, oral supplements with tablets of essential amino acids, and commercial preparations with a high content of amino acids.

Norton et al.[63] noted that their patients had a much better improvement of the skin rash (and restoration of plasma amino acids levels) with total parenteral nutrition solutions, and suggested, as discussed above, that the addition of carbohydrates facilitated the utilization of the infused amino acids.[85]

Local treatment of the skin rash will also be indicated, but it is difficult to point at a specific therapy. The anemia may need transfusion therapy.

## ACKNOWLEDGMENTS

Some of the studies reviewed here were supported by the Danish Medical Research Council, Daell-Fonden, and P. Carl Petersens Fond.

The clinical studies were performed in collaboration with Drs. Niels Bang Pedersen, Svein Helland, Stig Ingemansson and Gerda Frenz. Professor Lars-Inge Larsson performed the immunohistochemical and ultrastructural studies.

## REFERENCES

1. Becker SW, Kahn D, Rothman S: Cutaneous manifestations of internal malignant tumors. Arch Derm Syph 45:1069, 1942
2. Mallinson CN, Bloom SR, Warin AP, Salmon PR, Cox B: A glucagonoma syndrome. Lancet 2:1, 1974
3. Holst JJ: Glucagonomsyndromet. Ugeskr læg (Copenhagen) 137:2627, 1975

4. Binnick AN, Spencer SK, Landon Dennison W, Horton ES: Glucagonoma syndrome. Report of two cases and literature review. Arch Dermatol 113:749, 1977
5. Higgins GA, Recant L, Fischmann AB: The glucagonoma syndrome: Surgically curable diabetes. Am J Surg 137:142, 1979
6. Leichter SB: Clinical and metabolic aspects of glucagonoma Medicine 59:100, 1980
7. Stacpoole PW: The glucagonoma syndroma: Clinical features, diagnosis, and treatment. Endocrine Reviews 2:347, 1981
8. Bathena SJ, Higgins GA, Recant L: Glucagonoma and glucagonoma syndrome. In: Glucagon. Physiology, pathophysiology, and morphology of the pancreatic A-cells, eds. Unger RH, Orci L. New York, Elsevier 1981
9. Ruttman E, Kloppel G, Bommer G, Kiehn M, Heitz PU: Pancreatic glucagonoma with and without syndrome. Immunochemical study of 5 tumour cases and review of the literature. Virch Arch Abt A 388:51, 1980
10. Grimelius L, Hultquist GT, Stenkvist B: Cytological differentiation of asymptomatic pancreatic islet cell tumours in autopsy material. Virch. Arch. abt. A 365:275, 1975
11. Lomsky R, Langr F, Vortel V: Demonstration of glucagon in islet cell adenomas of the pancreas by immunofluorescent technic. Am J Clin Pathol 51:245, 1969
12. Warner TFCS, Block M, Hafez GR, Mack E, Lloyd RV, Bloom SR: Glucagonomas. Ultrastructure and immunocytochemistry. Cancer 51:1091, 1983
13. Bordi C, Ravazzola M, Baetens D, Gorden P, Unger RH, Orci L: A study of glucagon-omas by light and electron microscopy and immunofluorescence. Diabetes 28:925–936, 1979
14. Feiner H: Electron microscopy of neoplasms of pancreatic islet cells. J Dermatol Surg Oncol 4:751, 1978
15. Lubetzki J, Grupper Ch, Malbec D, et al: Une observation de glucagonome. 1—etude clinique, biologique, histologique, ultrastructurale et therapeutique. Nouv Presse Med 9:1565, 1980
16. von Schenck H, Thorell JI, Berg J, et al: Metabolic studies and glucagon gel filtration pattern before and after surgery in a case of glucagonoma syndrome. Acta Med Scand 205:155, 1979
17. Larsson LI: Endocrine Pancreatic Tumors. Hum Pathol 9:401, 1978
18. Larsson LI, Grimelius L, Håkanson R, et al: Mixed endocrine pancreatic tumors producing several peptide hormones. Am J Pathol 79:271, 1975
19. Ingemansson S, Holst J, Larsson LI, Lunderquist A: Localization of glucagonomas by catheterization of the pancreatic veins and with glucagon assay. Surg Gynecol Obstet 145:504, 1977
20. Larsson LI, Schwartz TW, Lundquist G, et al: Occurrence of human pancreatic poly-peptide in pancreatic endocrine tumors. Am J Pathol 85:675, 1976
21. Polak JM, Bloom SR, Adrian TE, et al: Pancreatic Polypeptide in insulinomas, gastrin-omas, vipomas and glucagonomas. Lancet 1:328, 1976
22. Wellbourn RB, Wood SM, Polak JM, Bloom SR: Pancreatic endocrine tumours. In: Gut hormones, eds: Bloom SR, Polak JM. Edinburgh, Churchill Livingstone 1981, pp 547
23. Tiengo A, Fedele D, Marchiori E, Nosadini R, Muggeo M: Suppression and stimula-tions mechanisms controlling glucagon secretion in a case of islet-cell tumor producing glucagon, insulin, and gastrin. Diabetes 25:408, 1976
24. Boden G, Owen OE, Rezvani I, et al: An islet cell carcinoma containing glucagon and insulin. Diabetes 26:128, 1977
25. Bloom SR, Polak JM, West AM: Somatostatin content of pancreatic endocrine tumors. Metabolism 27:1235, 1978

26. Belchetz PE, Brown CL, Makin HLJ, Trafford DJH, Mason AS, Bloom SR, Ratcliffe JG: ACTH, glucagon and gastrin production by a pancreatic islet cell carcinoma and its treatment. Clin Endocrinol 2:307, 1973

27. Hayashi M, Floyd JC, Pek S, Fajans SS: Insulin, proinsulin, glucagon, and gastrin in pancreatic tumors and in plasma of patients with organic hyperinsulinism. J Clin Endocrinol Metab 44:681, 1977

28. Wood SM, Bloom SR: Glucagon and gastrin secretion by a pancreatic tumour and its metastases. J Roy Soc Med 75:42, 1982

29. Ohneda A, Otsuki M, Fujiya H, et al: A malignant insulinoma transformed into a glucagonoma syndrome. Diabetes 28:962, 1979

30. Feurle GE, Helmstaedter V, Tischbirek K, et al: A multihormonal tumor of the pancreas producing neurotensin. Dig Dis Sci 26:1125, 1981

31. Vance JE, Stoll RW, Kitabchi AE, et al: Nesidioblastosis in familial andocrine adenomatosis. JAMA 207:1679, 1969

32. Croisier JC, Lehy T, Zeitoun P: A-2 cell pancreatic microadenomas in a case of multiple endocrine adenomatosis. Cancer 28:707, 1971

33. Croughs RJM, Hulsman HAM, Israel DE, et al: Glucagonoma as part of the polyglandular adenoma syndrome. Am J Med 52:690, 1972

34. Vance JE, Stoll RW, Kitabchi AE, et al: Familial nesidioblastosis as the predominant manifestation of multiple endocrine adenomatosis. Am J Med 52:211, 1972

35. Stacpoole PW, Jaspan J, Kasselberg AG, et al: A familial glucagonoma syndrome. Genetic, clinical and biochemical features. Am J Med 70:1017, 1981

36. Sibrack LA, Gouterman IH: Cutaneous manifestations of pancreatic diseases. Cutis 21:763, 1978

37. Rockl H, Metz J, Ackermann-Schopf C: Staphylodermia superficialis circinata. Die 5. obligate kutane Paraneoplasie. Der Hautartz 28:178, 1977

38. Unger RH, Lochner JV, Eisentraut AM: Identification of insulin and glucagon in a bronchogenic metastasis. J Clin Endocrinol 24:823, 1964

39. Hansen M, Hansen HH, Hirsch FR, et al: Hormonal polypeptides and amine metabolites in small cell carcinoma of the lung—with special reference to stage and subtypes. Cancer 45:1432, 1980

40. Roggli VL, Judge DM, McGavran MH: Duodenal glucagonoma: A case report. Hum Pathol 10:350, 1979

41. Gleeson MH, Bloom SR, Polak JM, et al: Endocrine tumour in kidney affecting small bowel structure, motility, and absorptive function. Gut 12:773–1971

42. Pavelic K, Popovic M: Insulin and glucagon secretion by renal adenocarcinoma. Cancer 48:98, 1981

43. Bloom SR: An enteroglucagon tumour. Gut 13:520, 1972

44. Holst JJ: Gut Glucagon, enteroglucagon, gut glucagonlike immunoreactivity, glicentin—current status. Gastroenterology 84:1602, 1983

45. Wilander E, Portela-Gomes G, Grimelius L, et al: Enteroglucagon and substance P-like immunoreactivity in argentaffin and argyrophil rectal carcinoids. Virch. Arch. B, Cell Pathol 25:117, 1977

46. Fiocca R, Capella C, Buffa R, et al: Glucagon-, glicentin-, and pancreatic polypeptide-like immunoreactivities in rectal carcinoids and related colorectal cells. Am J Pathol 100:81, 1980

47. Swenson KH, Amon RB, Hanifin JM: The glucagonoma syndrome. A distinctive cutaneous marker of systemic disease. Arch Dermatol 114:224, 1978

48. Boden G, Owen OE: Familial hyperglucagonemia—an autosomal dominant disorder. N Engl J Med 296:534, 1977

49. Helland S, Thorsen E, Holst JJ, Ingemansson S: Glukagonomsyndromet- nekrolytisk migrerende erythem. Tidsskr Nor Lægeforen 99:638, 1979
50. McGavran MH, Unger RH, Recant L, et al: A glucagon-secreting alpha-cell carcinoma of the pancreas. N Engl J Med 274:1408, 1966
51. Wilkinson DS: Necrolytic migratory erythema with carcinoma of the pancreas. Trans St John's Hosp Derm Soc 59:244, 1973
52. Sweet RD: A dermatosis specifically associated with a tumour of pancreatic alpha cells. Brit J Dermatol 90:301, 1974
53. Warin AP, Pegum JS: Necrolytic migratory erythema with carcinoma of pancreas. Proc roy Soc Med 67:24, 1974
54. Warin AP: Necrolytic Migratory Erythema with glucagon-secreting tumour of the pancreas. Proc Roy Soc Med 67:1008, 1974
55. Kahan RS, Perez-Figaredo MRA, Neimanis A: Necrolytic migratory erythema. Distinctive dermatosis of the glucagonoma syndrome. Arch Dermatol 113:792, 1977
56. Katz R, Fischmann AB, Galotto J, et al: Necrolytic migratory erythema, presenting as candidiasis, due to pancreatic glucagonoma. Cancer 44:558, 1979
57. Pedersen NB, Jonsson L, Holst JJ: Necrolytic migratory erythema and glucagon cell tumour of the pancreas: the glucagonoma syndrome. Acta Dermatovener (Stockholm) 56:391, 1976
58. Freedberg IM et al: Case record of the Mass General Hospital. N Engl J Med 292:1117, 1975
59. Weir GC, Horton ES, Aoki TT, et al: Secretion by glucagonomas of a possible glucagon precursor. J Clin Invest 59:325, 1977
60. Kessinger A, Lemon HM, Foley JF: The glucagonoma syndrome and its management. J Surg Oncol 9:419, 1977
61. Krebs A, Teuscher A, Armagni C: Syndrome de Glucagonome: Manifestations cutanees. Ann Dermatol Venerol (Paris) 105:637, 1978
62. Shupack JL, Berczeller PH, Stevens DM: The glucagonoma syndrome. J Dermatol Surg Oncol 4:242, 1978
63. Norton JA, Kahn CR, Schiebinger R, et al: Amino acid deficiency and the skin rash associated with glucagonoma syndrome. Ann Intern Med 91:213, 1979
64. Teuscher A, Studer PP, Krebs A, et al: Diabetesverlauf und klinisches Bild bei Glucagonom. Schweiz med Wschr 109:1273, 1979
65. Holst JJ, Helland S, Ingemansson S, et al: Functional studies in patients with the glucagonoma syndrome. Diabetologia 17:151, 1979
66. Berger M, Teuscher A, Halban P, et al: In vitro and in vivo studies onm glucagonoma tissue. Horm Metab Res 12:144, 1980
67. Montenegro F, Lawrence GD, Macon W, Pass C: Metastatic glucagonoma. Improvement after surgical debulking. Am J Surg 139:424, 1980
68. Takemiya M, Miyayama H, Takeya M, et al: A postmortem study of malignant glucagonoma with heart muscle hypertrophy, including chemical, histochemical, immunohistological, and ultrastructural observations. Hum Pathol 12:988, 1981
69. Prinz RA, Badrinath K, Banerji M, et al: Operative and chemotherapeutic management of malignant glucagon-producing tumors. Surgery 90:713, 1981
70. Hallengren B, Dymling JF, Manhem P, et al: Unsuccessful DTIC-treatment of a patient with glucagonoma syndrome. Acta Med Scand, 213:317, 1983
71. Linnestad P, Myrvang B, Ritland S, et al: Glucagonproduserende tumor i pancreas. Tidskr Nor Lægeforen 103:1520, 1983
72. Marliss EB, Aoki TT, Unger RH, et al: Glucagon levels and metabolic effects in fasting man. J Clin Invest 49:2256, 1970

73. Fitzpatrick GF, Meguid MM, Gitlitz PH, Brennan MF: Glucagon infusion in normal man: effects on 3-methylhistidine excretion and plasma amino acids. Metabolism 26:477, 1977

74. Wolfe BM, Culebras JM, Aoki TT, et al: The effects of glucagon on protein metabolism in normal man. Surgery 86:248, 1979

75. Liljenquist JE, Lewis SB, Cherrington AD, et al: Effects of pharmacologic hyperglucagonemia on plasma amino acid concentrations in normal and diabetic man. Metabolism 30:1195, 1981

76. Brodan V, Brodanova M, Andel M, Kuhn E: The effect of glucagon on free plasma amino acids in cirrhotics and healthy controls Acta hepato-gastroenterol 25:23, 1978

77. Muller WA, Berger M, Suter P, et al: Glucagon immunoreactivities and amino acid profile in plasma of duodenopancreatectomized patients. J Clin Invest 63:820, 1979

78. Boden G, Master RW, Rezvani I, et al: Glucagon deficiency and hyperaminoacidemia after total pancreatectomy. J Clin Invest 65:706, 1980

79. Muller WA, Cuppers HJ, Zimmerman-Telschow H, et al: Aminoacids and lipoproteins in plasma of duodenopancreatectomized patients: effects of glucagon in physiological amounts. Eur J Clin Invest 13:141, 1983

80. Holst JJ: Glucagon—how to prove its role in amino acid metabolism. Eur J Clin Invest 13:107, 1983

81. Hennington UM, Caroe E, Derbes V: Kwashiorkor. Report of four cases from Louisiana. Arch Dermatol 78:157, 1958

82. Adams EB, Scragg JN, Naidoe BT: Observations on the etiology and treatment of anemia in kwashiorkor. Brit J Med 2:451, 1967

83. Truswell AS, Leadsky C, Wettmann W: Are the skin lesions of Kwashiorkor pellagrous? S Afr Med J 36:965, 1967

84. Marynick SP, Fagadau WR, Duncan LA: Malignant glucagonoma Syndrome: Response to chemotherapy. Ann Int Med 93:453, 1980

85. Wolfe BM, Culebras JM, Sim AJW, et al: Substrate interaction in intravenous feeding: comparative effects of carbohydrate and fat on amino acid utilization in fasting man. Ann Surg 186:518, 1977

86. Barber SG, Hamer FD: Skin rash in patient receiving glucagon. Lancet II:1138, 1976

87. Ferranini E, DeFronzo RA, Sherwin RS: Transient hepatic response to glucagon in man: role of insulin and hyperglycemia. Am J Physiol 242:E73, 1982

88. Sacca L, Eigler N, Goldberg D, Walefsky M: Hormonal interactions in the regulation of blood glucose. Rec Prog Horm Res 35:501, 1979

89. Gossner VW, Korting GW: Metastasierendes Inselzellkarzinom vom A-zelltyp bei einem Fall von Pemphigus Foliaceus mit Diabetes renalis. Dtschr med Wschr 85:434, 1960

90. Church RE, Crane WAJ: A cutaneous syndrome associated with islet-cell carcinoma of the pancreas. Br J Dermatol 79:284, 1967

91. Danforth DN, Triche T, Doppman JL, et al: Elevated plasma proglucagon-like component with a glucagon-secreting tumor. Effect of streptozotocin. N Engl J Med 295:242, 1976

92. Soler NG, Oates GD, Malins JM: Glucagonoma syndrome in a young man. Proc roy Soc Med 69:429, 1976

93. Lefebvre J, Lelievre G, Dalle-Furnari MA, et al: Glucagonoma avec acidocetose diabetique. Une observation. Diabete Metab (Paris) 8:191, 1982

94. Domen RE, Shaffer MB, Finke J, Et al: The glucagonoma syndrome: report of a case. Arch Intern Med 140:262, 1980

95. Kahn D, Bhatena SJ, Recant L, Rivier J: Use of somatostatin and somatostatin analogs in a patient with a glucagonoma. J Clin Endocrinol Metab 53:543, 1981

96. Boden G, Wilson RM, Owen OE: Effects of chronic glucagon excess on hepatic metabolism. Diabetes 27:643, 1978

97. Nankervis A, Proietto J, Ng KW, et al: The metabolic effects of chronic hyperglucagonemia. Clin Endocrinol 15:325, 1981

98. Condon JR: Glucagon and blood sugar. N Engl J Med 295:451, 1976

99. Cherrington AD, Diamond MP, Green DR, Williams PE: Evidence for an intrahepatic contribution to the waning effect of glucagon on glucose production in the conscious dog. Diabetes 31:917, 1982

100. Fukushima H, Yamaguchi K, Uzawa H, et al: A case with glucagonoma syndrome—endocrine and metabolic studies. Endocrinol Japon 28:111, 1981

101. Lightman SL, Bloom SR: Cure of insulin-dependent diabetes mellitus by removal of a glucagonoma. Brit Med J 1:367, 1974

102. Beltzer-Garelli E, Cesarini JP, Cywiner-Golenzer Ch, et al: Lesions cutanees revelatrices d'un glucagonome. Sem Hop Paris 56:579, 1980

103. Khandekar JD, Oyer D, Miller HJ, Vick NA: Neurologic involvement in glucagonoma syndrome. Response to combination chemotherapy with 5-fluorouracil and streptozotocin. Cancer 44:2014, 1979

104. Naets JP, Guns M: Inhibitory effect of glucagon on erythropoiesis. Blood 55:997, 1980

105. Sturner WQ: Sudden death from non-insulin secreting islet cell tumor of the pancreas ("glucagonoma"). Hum Pathol 3:113, 1972

106. Villar HV, Johnson DG, Lynch PJ, et al: Pattern of immunoreactive glucagon in portal, arterial and peripheral plasma before and after removal of glucagonoma. Am J Surg 141:148, 1981

107. Beutner EH, Jordon RE, Chorzelski TP: The immunopathology of pemphigus and bullous pemphigoid. J Investigative Dermatol 51:63, 1968

108. Prasad AS: Clinical, biochemical, and pharmacological role of zinc. Ann Rev Pharmacol Toxicol 20:393, 1979

109. Kay RG, Tasman-Jones C, Pybus J, et al: A syndrome of acute zinc deficiency during total parental alimentation in man. Ann Surg 183:331, 1976

110. Tasman-Jones C, Kay RG: Zinc deficiency and skin lesions. New Engl J Med 293:830, 1975

111. Lyell A: Toxic epidermal necrolysis (the scalded skin syndrome): A reappraisal. Brit J Dermatol 100:69, 1979

112. Cantwell AR, Martz W. Idiopathic bullae in diabetics. Arch Dermatol 96:42, 1967

113. Allen GE, Hadden DR: Bullous lesions of the skin in diabetes (bullosis diabeticorum). Brit J Dermatol. 82:216, 1970

114. Dobozy A, Husz S, Schneider I, Szabo E: Bullous dermatosis associated with latent diabetes. Dermatologica 144:283, 1972

115. Goodenberger DM, Lawley TJ, Strober W, et al: Necrolytic migratory erythema without glucagonoma. Arch Dermatol 115:1429, 1979

116. Doyle JA, Schroetter AL, Rogers RS: Hyperglucagonemia and necrolytic migratory erythema in cirrhosis-possible pseudoglucagonoma syndrome. Brit J Dermatol 100:581, 1979

117. Thivolet J, Perrot CL, Hermier CL, Pellerat J: Erytheme cutanee migrateur avec necrose epidermique superficielle au cours d'une pancreatite chronique. Bull Soc franc Derm Syph 81:415, 1974

118. Melani F, Ryan WG, Rubenstein AH, Steiner DF: Proinsulin secretion by a pancreatic beta-cell adenoma. Proinsulin and C-peptide secretion. N Engl J Med 283:713, 1970
119. Kitabchi AE: Proinsulin and C-peptide: A review. Metabolism 26:547, 1977
120. Holst JJ, Bang Pedersen N: Glucagon producing tumors of the pancreas. Acta Endocrinol (Kbh) suppl 199:379, 1975
121. Holst JJ: Molecular heterogeneity of glucagon in normal subjects and in patients with glucagon-producing tumours. Diabetologia 24:359, 1983
122. Valverde I, Lemon HM, Kessinger A, Unger RH: Distribution of plasma glucagon immunoreactivity in a patient with suspected glucagonoma. J Clin Endocrin Metab 42:804, 1976
123. Recant L, Perrino PV, Bhatena SJ, et al: Plasma immunoreactive glucagon fractions in four cases of glucagonoma: Increased "Large glucagon-immunoreactivity." Diabetologia 12:319, 1976
124. Stefan Y, Ravazzola M, Orci L: Primitive islets contain two populations of cells with differing glucagon immunoreactivity. Diabetes 30:192, 1981
125. Bell GI, Santerre RF, Mullenbach GT: Hamster preproglucagon contains the sequence of glucagon and two related peptides. Nature 302:716, 1983
126. Lubetzki J, Grupper CH, Gmalbec D, et al: Une observation de glucagonome. II: Exploration hormonale. Nouv Presse Med 9:1623, 1980
127. Dagget PR, Goodburn EA. Kurtz AB, Le Quesne LP, Morris DV, Nabarro JDN, Raphael MJ: Is preoperative localisation of insulinomas necessary? Lancet 1:483, 1981
128. Ghosh BC, Mojab K, Esfahani F, et al: Role of angiography in the diagnosis of pancreatic neoplasms. Am J Surg 138:675, 1979
129. Cho KJ, Wilcox CW, Reuter SR: Glucagon-producing islet cell tumour of the pancreas. Am J Roentgenol 129:159, 1977
130. Modlin IM: Endocrine tumors of the pancreas. Surg Gyn Obstet 149:751, 1979
131. Friesen SR: Tumors of the endocrine pancreas. N Engl J Med 306:580, 1982
132. Ingemansson S, Lunderquist A, Holst J: Selective catheterization of the pancreatic vein for radioimmunoassay in glucagonsecreting carcinoma of the pancreas. Radiology 119:555, 1976
133. Molinie C, Naudan P, Daly JP, et al: Glucagonome: Survie de neuf annees apres exerese. Nouv Presse Med 10:177, 1981
134. Murray-Lyon IM, Eddleston ALWF, Williams R, et al: Treatment of multiple hormone producing malignant islet cell tumour with streptozotocin. Lancet 2:895, 1968
135. Broder LE, Carter SK: Pancreatic islet cell carcinoma. II. Results of streptozotocin treatment in 52 patients. Ann Int Med 79:108, 1973
136. Strauss GM, Weitzman SA, Aoki TT: Dimethyltriazenoimidazole carboxamide therapy of malignant glucagonoma. Ann Int Med 90:57, 1979
137. Ruffner BW: Chemotherapy for malignant Zollinger-Ellison tumors. Arch Int Med. 136:1032, 1976
138. Duncan LA, Marynick SP: Glucagonoma and Dacarbazine. Ann Intern Med 97:930, 1982

# 4 | Somatostatinoma

*Guenther Boden*
*Ryushi Shimoyama*

## INTRODUCTION

In 1969, Krulich and McCann first reported that crude hypothalamic extracts inhibited the release of growth hormone from rat pituitaries in vitro.[1] The active principle responsible for this effect was isolated, purified, sequenced, synthesized, and named somatostatin by investigators at the Salk Institute in the years between 1972 and 1974.[2-4] The availability of synthetic somatostatin led in rapid sequence to the discovery of its inhibitory actions on the release of many polypeptide hormones and to the development of sensitive and specific radioimmunoassays for its measurement. It was soon discovered that somatostatin was present in high concentrations not only in the central and peripheral nervous system but also in the intestinal tract and the pancreas where it is synthesized and released from specific D cells in the pancreatic islets and the intestinal mucosa and from neurons in the central nervous system (for review see Ref. 5).

Radioimmunological determination of somatostatin-like-immunoreactivity (SLI) in biological fluids also led to the recognition of abnormalities in somatostatin synthesis and secretion. For instance, it was found that the pancreatic islet cell content of somatostatin was increased in streptozotocin diabetic mice and rats[6,7] and that there was an apparent increase in D cells in islets of patients with insulin-dependent diabetes mellitus.[8] In 1977, Ganda[9] and Larsson[10] independently reported the first two cases of somatostatinoma (i.e., tumors containing and/or secreting excessive amounts of somatostatin). On the basis of these reports, Unger tentatively proposed a clinical somatostatinoma syndrome consisting of mild diabetes, gallbladder disease, weight loss, and anemia.[11] Diarrhea, steatorrhea, and hypochlorhydria became additional features as more cases were discovered.[12,13]

For the purpose of this review, we have defined somatostatinomas as tumors in which there was evidence of abnormally high concentrations of tumor somatostatin or D cells or of abnormally elevated concentrations of plasma SLI. Using this definition, we have collected 20 cases[9,10,12-25] reported in the literature between 1977 and 1983. Some of those cases had the clinical somatostatinoma syndrome while others did not. In selecting these cases, we have focused our attention on tumors originating from the gastrointestinal tract. Somatostatin-secreting tumors originating outside the GI tract, however, are also discussed briefly.

## CLINICAL FEATURES (TABLE 4-1)

### Age and Sex of Patients with Somatostatinoma

The mean age of the 20 patients was 51.2 years, with a range from 26 to 84 years. Thirteen of the 20 patients were between 40 and 60 years old, only 4 were younger than 40 years and only 3 were older than 60 years (Fig. 4-1). Clearly, somatostatinoma appears to be a disease of the middle age similar to other islet cell tumors such as insulinoma[26] and glucagonoma.[27]

Eleven of the 20 patients were female, 9 were male, suggesting equal sex distribution. Similarly, no significant sex differences were found in 234 cases of insulinoma.[26]

**Table 4-1.** Clinical Features of Somatostatinoma Patients

| Case | Authors (Ref. No.) | Age/Sex | Diabetes | Gallbladder Disease | Diarrhea |
|------|--------------------|---------|----------|---------------------|----------|
| 1 | Ganda et al (9) | 46/F | yes | yes | — |
| 2 | Larsson et al (10) | 55/F | yes | yes | yes |
| 3 | Pipeleers et al (14) | 56/F | yes | yes | — |
| 4 | Galmiche et al (15) | 70/F | yes | yes | yes |
| 5 | Kaneko et al (13) | 26/M | — | — | — |
| 6 | Krejs et al (12) | 52/M | yes | yes | yes |
| 7 | Wright et al (16) | 33/F | no | yes | — |
| 8 | Penman et al (17) | 36/M | yes | — | — |
| 9 | Axelrod et al (18) | 54/F | yes | yes | yes |
| 10 | Lowry et al (19) | 50/M | yes | yes | — |
| 11 | Stacpoole (20) | 36/F | yes | yes | yes |
| 12 | Stacpoole (20) | 53/M | — | — | — |
| 13 | Alumets et al (21) | 55/F | — | yes | — |
| 14 | Cantor et al (22) | 49/F | no | yes | — |
| 15 | Kovacs et al (23) | 54/M | yes | — | — |
| 16 | Fujiya et al (24) | 51/M | no | — | — |
| 17 | Pipeleers (25) | 54/M | yes | — | — |
| 18 | Pipeleers (25) | 47/M | no | — | — |
| 19 | Pipeleers (25) | 84/F | yes** | yes | — |
| 20 | Pipeleers (25) | 63/F | no | yes | — |

\* Metastatic involvement of skin, liver, kidneys, ovaries, adrenals and thyroid
\*\* Mild glucose intolerance

**Table 4-1** (*Continued*)

| | | | SLI | | | |
| Steat-<br>orrhea | Hypochlor-<br>hydria | Weight<br>Loss | Plasma<br>(ng/ml) | Tumor<br>(ng/mg) | Tumor<br>Site | Metastases |
|---|---|---|---|---|---|---|
| — | — | yes | — | 301 | P. Head | Lymph<br>Node |
| yes | yes | — | 107 | — | P. Head | Liver |
| yes | — | — | 30.8 | — | P. Head | Liver |
| yes | yes | yes | 9.0 | 134 | P. Head | Liver |
| — | no | — | — | 2.2 | Duodenum | — |
| yes | — | yes | 13.0 | 5000 | P. Whole<br>Organ | Liver |
| — | — | — | 16.8 | 54 | P. Head | Liver, nodes |
| — | — | — | 0.16 | 5.0 | P. Tail | — |
| — | — | — | 0.9 | 1.37 | P. Head | Liver* |
| yes | — | yes | 20 | — | P. Head | Liver |
| — | — | — | 0.16 | 0.006 | P. Tail | Local Nodes |
| — | — | — | 0.16 | 0.045 | Duodenum | Local Nodes |
| — | — | — | — | — | Jejunum | Local Nodes |
| — | — | yes | — | — | Duodenum | No |
| — | — | yes | — | — | P. Tail | Liver |
| — | — | — | — | 0.6 | — | Liver, Local<br>Nodes |
| — | — | yes | 5.2 | 72 | P. Head | Liver |
| — | — | — | 0.5 | 0.56 | P. Head | — |
| — | — | — | 12.5 | 0.6 | P. Head | Liver |
| — | — | — | 0.6 | 1.2 | P. Head | Liver |

## Plasma SLI

Plasma SLI was determined in 14 of the 20 patients. Mean SLI concentration was 15.5 ng/ml (range 0.16 to 107 ng/ml). Some of those determinations, however, were done with unextracted plasma which is now known to give falsely elevated results. In 13 cases, plasma SLI values from somatostatinoma patients were compared with control values established in the same laboratories. Mean plasma SLI concentrations in patients with somatostatinoma was 50 times higher than normal (range 1–250 times). Two of these 13 cases, however, had normal and 2 others had only slightly elevated SLI concentrations (1.2 times normal).

## Heterogeneity of Plasma SLI

Molecular heterogeneity of SLI in plasma was reported in 6 cases. SLI eluting in the area of the somatostatin marker (MW 1600 daltons) was present in all 6 and represented the major fraction in 3 cases. SLI with an apparent molecular weight of between 3000 and 4000 daltons was found in 5 cases and represented the major fraction in 1. SLI eluting with an apparent molecular weight of between 6000 and 7000 or 10,000 and 15,000 daltons was present in 6 cases and represented the largest fraction in one. SLI with an apparent molecular weight of greater than 30,000 daltons was reported in 2 cases. Thus, the plasma of many patients with somatostatinoma contained 3–4 different molecular forms of SLI, specifically

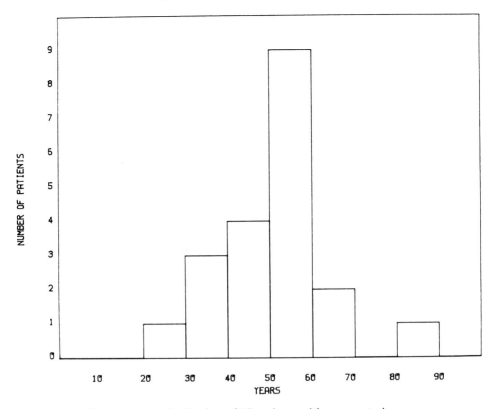

**Fig. 4-1.**  Age distribution of 20 patients with somatostatinoma.

of SLI fractions with apparent molecular weights of 1600, 3000–4000, 6000–15,000 and greater than 30,000 daltons. Some of these molecular fractions may be somatostatin precursors. Release into the circulation of abnormally large amounts of high molecular weight forms of polypeptide hormones is a characteristic feature of endocrine tumors, including insulinomas and glucagonomas. Presence of an increased percentage of proinsulin in the circulation has been used as a diagnostic marker for insulinoma. Conceivably, measurement of higher molecular weight SLI in plasma may in the future become a useful tool in the diagnosis of somatostatinoma.

## Diabetes Mellitus

Eleven of 20 cases had diabetes mellitus, a 12th case was described as having mild glucose intolerance. Absence of a family history of diabetes was specifically mentioned in 2 cases. In all instances, the diabetes was relatively mild and could be controlled with diet and/or hypoglycemic agents or with small doses of insulin. In 1 patient,[18] however, ketonemia (total serum ketone body concentration of ap-

One patient had widespread metastatic disease to the skin, liver, kidneys, ovaries, adrenal and thyroid glands. Thus, in approximately 80% of the cases, metastatic disease was present at the time of diagnosis. This is similar to the high incidence of malignancy in glucagonoma[27] and in gastrinoma,[38] but it is distinctly different from the low incidence of malignant insulinoma.[26] The high prevalence of metastatic disease in somatostatinoma may also be a consequence of late diagnosis.

## Microscopic Appearance

On light microscopy, most tumors appeared as well differentiated islet cell or carcinoid tumors. Some showed a mixed picture consisting of separate zones of differentiated and anaplastic cells. In the differentiated areas, cells were arranged in lobular or acinar patterns separated by fibrovascular stroma. Less well differentiated areas consisted of sheets of cells interrupted by fibrous septa.

Electron microscopic examination was performed on 9 tumors. In 8, the secretory granules were reported to have the typical appearance of D cell granules, while in one case they were described as atypical. This is somewhat unusual, inasmuch as the electron microscopic appearance of secretory granules in malignant islet cells is frequently atypical. Immunocytochemical testing was performed on tissues of 15 tumors. Most of the antisera used recognized the C terminal end of the somatostatin molecule. All 15 tumors showed presence of SLI containing cells. In addition, there was immunological evidence for the presence of cells containing insulin in 5 tumors, calcitonin in 4, gastrin in 2 and VIP, ACTH, $PGE_2$ and substance P in 1 tumor each. However, in the tumors with multiple hormones SLI containing cells represented the large majority of all immune staining cells in all but 2. The 2 exceptions,[24,25] both presented with hypoglycemia, were diagnosed as insulinomas. From 1 of these 2 cases, only metastatic tissue was available for immunecytochemical testing; it showed B cells representing 30–40%, D cells 20–30% and G cells 25–35% of all immune staining cells. The pancreatic tumor from the second case reacted weakly with both SLI and insulin antibodies.

## Tumor SLI Content

Information of SLI tumor content was available in 14 cases. In 1 additional case, tumor SLI content was described as large. The mean SLI tumor content was 398 ng/mg of wet weight with a range from 0.006 to 5000 ng/mg of wet weight. In 10 of the 14 cases in which tumor SLI content was compared with SLI content of normal pancreatic tissue, the SLI tumor content was an average of 1163 times greater than normal (range: 9 to 7812 times).

## Heterogeneity of Tumor SLI

SLI extracts from 10 somatostatinomas were gel filtrated. In 7, the predominant molecular form of SLI was similar in size to the synthetic 1600 dalton tetradecapeptide. Three tumors contained, in addition, SLI material with an apparent molecular weight of between 10 and 15,000 daltons. There is evidence to suggest[39] that the biosynthesis of somatostatin proceeds via a 12,000 dalton pro-somatostatin. Therefore, it is likely that the 10,000–15,000 dalton SLI component found in somatostatinomas may represent a somatostatin precursor.

## Tumor Content of Other Hormones

Radioimmunological evidence for the presence of hormones other than SLI in concentrations equal or greater than normal was reported in 6 tumors. Two tumor extracts contained insulin, 1 contained insulin and glucagon, 1 contained substance P and VIP, and 1 tumor extract each contained calcitonin and motilin. Therefore, the evidence derived from radioimmunoassays of tumor extracts and from immunecytochemical staining techniques indicated that somatostatinoma, as other islet cell tumors, frequently contain more than 1 hormone.

# DIAGNOSIS

All somatostatinomas in this series were found more or less accidentally. In 5 cases a pancreatic or duodenal mass was seen during cholecystectomy. In a 6th case, a duodenal tumor was discovered during resection of a pheochromocytoma. In the remaining cases, the tumors were found either during exploratory laporotomy or during upper gastrointestinal x-ray studies, CAT scans, or ultrasound or endoscopic studies performed because of various symptoms including unexplained abdominal pain, melena, hematemesis, persistent diarrhea, or in search of insulinomas or ACTH secreting tumors. Once found, the tumors were identified as somatostatinoma by demonstration of elevated tissue concentrations of SLI and/ or prevalence of D cells by immunocytochemistry or by the demonstration of elevated plasma SLI concentrations. Thus, the events leading to the diagnosis of somatostatinoma have occurred in reverse order. In other islet cell tumors, the clinical symptoms and signs usually suggest the diagnosis which is then established by the demonstration of diagnostically elevated blood hormone levels following which efforts are undertaken to localize the tumors. It can be expected that the same sequence of diagnostic procedures will be followed in the future for the diagnosis of somatostatinoma mainly for two reasons. (1) The increasing familiarity of physicians with the clinical somatostatinoma syndrome (Table 4-2). This symptom complex, while not pathognomonic, is nevertheless sufficiently characteristic for somatostatinoma to suggest the correct diagnosis. (2) The greater availability of reliable radioimmunoassays for the determination of SLI in blood. Presently these assays are complicated by the need for cumbersome extraction procedures and are not readily available.

Present evidence suggests that the clinical somatostatinoma syndrome develops at advanced stages of the disease when the tumors have grown large and have metastasized in many cases. Early diagnosis is, therefore, of utmost importance.

**Table 4-2.** The Clinical Somatostatinoma Syndrome

| |
|---|
| Diabetes mellitus (nonketotic) |
| Gallbladder Disease |
| Diarrhea/Steatorrhea |
| Hypochlorhydria |
| Weight Loss |
| Anemia |
| Elevated Plasma SLI |

The diagnosis of somatostatinoma at a time when blood SLI concentrations are normal or only marginally elevated, however, will require reliable provocative tests. Increases in plasma SLI concentrations have been reported in 4 cases, each after intravenous infusion of tolbutamide and arginine. Decreases in SLI concentrations have been observed in 2 cases after intravenous infusion of diazoxide. Arginine is a well established stimulant for normal D cells and thus is unlikely to differentiate between normal and supranormal somatostatin secretion. The same may be true for diazoxide, which has been shown to decrease SLI secretion from normal dog pancreas as well as in patients with somatostatinoma.[40] Tolbutamide has been found to stimulate SLI release from normal dog and rat pancreas[40,41] but Pipeleers[25] found no change in circulating SLI concentrations in three normal human subjects after IV injection of 1 g of tolbutamide. At present, therefore, tolbutamide appears to be a candidate for a provocative agent useful in the diagnosis of somatostatinoma. Clearly, however, its reliability will have to be established in a greater number of patients and controls. Until then, it may be necessary to measure plasma SLI concentrations during routine workups for postprandial dyspepsia and gallbladder disorders as suggested by Krejs,[12] inasmuch as these symptoms appear to be very early signs of somatostatinomas.

## TREATMENT AND OUTCOME

Twelve patients underwent surgery. Of those, 8 patients had total or partial pancreatectomy with or without extirpation of liver metastases or hepatic lobectomy. The 4 patients with duodenal or jejunal tumors had duodenectomy or jejunectomy. Four patients received chemotherapy and 2 patients had surgery and chemotherapy. Chemotherapy consisted of streptozotocin alone in three patients. One patient received streptozotocin together with 5 fluorouracil, dicarbazine, and doxorubicin. Another patient received 5 fluorouracil and diazoxide and in 1 patient the type of chemotherapy was not specified. Two patients received no specific treatment. Eight of the 20 patients died at intervals ranging from 1 week to 14 months after diagnosis. Two patients died in hypoglycemic coma, the remaining one as a result of metastatic disease. Twelve patients were alive from 6 months to 5 years after diagnosis.

# SOMATOSTATIN-CONTAINING TUMORS OUTSIDE
# THE GI TRACT

Somatostatin has been found in many tissues outside the GI tract. Prominent among those are the hypothalamic and extrahypothalamic regions of the brain, the peripheral nervous system including the sympathetic noradrenergic ganglia, and the C cells of the thyroid gland. Not surprisingly, therefore, high concentrations of somatostatin have been found in tumors originating from these tissues. Sano et al. and Saito et al. reported 7 patients with medullary carcinoma of the thyroid (MTC) who had high basal plasma SLI concentrations and high tumor SLI concentrations.[42,43] In addition, Roos et al.[44] reported elevated (136 to 6150 pg/ ml) plasma SLI concentrations in 3 of 7 patients with MTC and high tissue SLI concentrations (60–9200 pg/mg) in 3 of 5 MTC tumors. Fractionation of tumor tissue and plasma SLI revealed SLI peaks corresponding to apparent molecular weights of about 1600 and 10,000 daltons. Some but not all of these patients exhibited the clinical somatostatinoma syndrome.

Elevated plasma SLI concentrations have also been reported in 4 of 26 patients with small cell lung cancer.[44] Five of 9 of these cancers contained high concentrations of SLI (14–441 pg/mg). Ghose et al.[45] reported another case of a metastatic bronchial oat cell carcinoma causing Cushing syndrome, diabetes, diarrhea, steatorrhea, anemia and weight loss, and a plasma SLI concentration which was 20 times greater than normal. Pheochromocytomas[46] and catecholamine producing extra-adrenal paragangliomas[47] are other examples of endocrine tumors producing and secreting somatostatin in addition to other hormonally active substances.

# SUMMARY

Most of the 20 somatostatinomas were large, solitary tumors. Seventy-five percent were located in the pancreas and 20% were found in the duodenum or jejunum. At the time of diagnosis, 80% had metastasized to the liver and/or to regional lymph nodes. Somatostatinomas contained large amounts of two molecular forms of somatostatin. One was authentic somatostatin (molecular weight 1600 daltons). The other had an apparent molecular weight of between 10,000 and 15,000 and may have been a somatostatin precursor. Several somatostatinomas contained in addition other hormones including insulin, glucagon, gastrin, VIP, calcitonin, substance P, and motilin. The peak age incidence of somatostatinoma was in the fifth decade. Males and females were afflicted equally. Clinical features commonly observed in patients with somatostatinoma were diabetes mellitus, gallbladder disease, diarrhea and steatorrhea, hypochlorhydria, weight loss, anemia, and elevated plasma SLI concentrations. This complex of signs and symptoms has been named the "Clinical Somatostatinoma Syndrome." Approximately ½ of all patients with somatostatinoma had other endocrinopathies including insulinoma, gastrinoma, Cushing's Syndrome, pheochromocytoma, and goiter. In the past, most somatostatinomas were discovered accidentally, many during cholecystectomy. It is hoped that in the future greater recognition of the clinical somatostatinoma syndrome and greater availability of radioimmunoassays for the determination of SLI in plasma will lead to earlier diagnosis of this disorder. Twelve patients had surgical treatment, four chemotherapy and 2 surgery plus chemotherapy. The malignant nature of the disorder is underlined by the fact that 8 of the 20 patients died at intervals ranging from 1 week to 14 months after diagnosis.

## ACKNOWLEDGMENTS

Supported by USPHS Grants AM 190397 and 5M01–RR349. We thank Mrs. Vickie Fields for typing the manuscript.

## REFERENCES

1. Krulich L, McCann S: Effect of GH-releasing factor and GH-inhibiting factor on the release and concentration of GH in pituitaries incubated *in vitro*. Endocrinology 85:319, 1969
2. Brazeau P, Vale W, Burgus R, et al: Hypothalamic peptide that inhibits the secretion of immunoreactive pituitary growth hormone. Science 179:77, 1973
3. Burgus R, Ling N, Butcher M, et al: Primary structure of somatostatin, a hypothalamic peptide that inhibits the secretion of pituitary growth hormone. Proc Natl Acad Sci 70:684, 1973
4. Rivier JEF: Somatostatin. Total solid phase synthesis. J Am Chem Soc 96:2986, 1974
5. Guillemin R, Gerich JE: Somatostatin: Physiological and clinical significance. Ann Rev Med 27:379, 1976
6. Patel YC, Cameron DP: Somatostatin: widespread abnormality in tissues of spontaneously diabetic mice. Science 198:930, 1977
7. Patel YC, Cameron DP, Bankier A, et al: Changes in somatostatin concentration in pancreas and other tissues of streptozotocin diabetic rats. Endocrinology 103:917, 1978
8. Orci L, Baetens D, Rufener C, et al: Hypertrophy and hyperplasia of somatostatin-containing D-cells in diabetes. Proc Natl Acad Sci 73:1338, 1976
9. Ganda OP, Weir GC, Soeldner JS et al: 'Somatostatinoma': A somatostatin-containing tumor of the endocrine pancreas. N Engl J Med 296:963, 1977
10. Larsson L.-I, Holst JJ, Kühl C, et al: Pancreatic somatostatinoma. Clinical features and physiological implications. Lancet i:666, 1977
11. Unger RH: Somatostatinoma. N Engl J Med 296:998, 1977
12. Krejs GJ, Orci L, Conlon JM, et al: Somatostatinoma syndrome. N Engl J Med 301:285, 1979
13. Kaneko H, Yanaihara N, Ito S, et al: Somatostatinoma of the duodenum. Cancer 44:2273, 1979
14. Pipeleers D, Somers G, Gepts W, et al: Plasma pancreatic hormone levels in a case of somatostatinoma: Diagnostic and therapeutic implications. J Clin Endocrinol Metab 49:572, 1979
15. Galmiche JP, Chayvialle JA, Dubois PM et al: Calcitonin-producing pancreatic somatostatinoma. Gastroenterology 78:1577, 1980
16. Wright J, Abolfathi A, Penman E, et al: Pancreatic somatostatinoma presenting with hypoglycemia. Clin Endocrinol 12:603, 1980

17. Penman E, Lowry PJ, Wass JAH, et al: Molecular forms of somatostatin in normal subjects and in patients with pancreatic somatostatinoma. Clin Endocrinol 12:611, 1980

18. Axelrod L, Bush MA, Hirsch HJ, et al: Malignant Somatostatinoma: Clinical features and metabolite studies. J Clin Endocrinol Metab 52:886, 1981

19. Lowry SF, Burt ME, Brennan MF: Glucose turnover and gluconeogenesis in a patient with somatostatinoma. Surgery 89:309, 1981

20. Stacpoole PW, Kasselberg AG, Berelowitz M, et al: Somatostatinoma syndrome: does a clinical entity exist: Acta Endocrinologica 102:80, 1983

21. Alumets J, Ekelund G, Hakanson R, et al: Jejunal endocrine tumour composed of somatostatin and gastrin cells and associated with duodenal ulcer disease. Virchows Arch A Path Anat and Histol 378:17, 1978

22. Cantor AM, Rigby CC, Beck PP et al: Neurofibromatosis, phaeochromocytoma, and somatostatinoma. British Med J 285:1618, 1982

23. Kovacs K, Horvath E, Ezrin C, et al: Immunoreactive somatostatin in pancreatic islet-cell carcinoma accompanied by ectopic A.C.T.H. syndrome. Lancet 1:1365, 1977

24. Fujiya H, Kawabu A, Yanaihara N, et al: Malignant insulino-gastrino-somatostatinoma. Horumon to Rinsho 26:591, 1978 (In Japanese)

25. Pipeleers D, Couturier E, Gepts W, et al: Five cases of somatostatinoma: Clinical heterogeneity and diagnostic usefulness of basal and tolbutamide-induced hypersomatostatinemia. J Clin Endocrinol Metab 56:1236, 1983

26. Crain EL, Jr, Thorn GW: Functioning pancreatic islet cell adenomas. Medicine 28:427, 1949

27. Bhathena SJ, Higgins GA, Recant L: Glucagonoma and glucagonoma syndrome. In: Glucagon, eds. Unger RH, Orci L. Elsevier North Holland Inc. New York, 1981, p. 413

28. Mandarino L, Stenner D, Blanchard W, et al: Selective effects of somatostatin-14, -25 and -28 on *in vitro* insulin and glucagon secretion. Nature 291:76, 1981

29. Gerich JE, Lovinger R, Grodsky GM: Inhibition by somatostatin of glucagon and insulin release from the perfused rat pancreas in response to arginine, isoproterenol and theophylline: evidence for a preferential effect on glucagon secretion. Endocrinology 96:749, 1975

30. Efendic S, Claro A, Luft R: Studies on the mechanism of somatostatin action on insulin release. III. Effect of somatostatin on arginine induced release of insulin and glucagon in man and perfused rat pancreas. Acta Endocrinol (Copenh) 81:753, 1976

31. Hermansen K, Schwartz TW: Differential sensitivity to somatostatin of pancreatic poly-peptide, glucagon and insulin secretion from the isolated perfused canine pancreas. Metabolism 28:1229, 1979

32. Creutzfeldt W, Lankisch PG, Folsch UR: Hemmung der Secretin und Cholezystokinin-Pankreozymin-induzierten Saft und Enzymsecretion des Pancreas und der Gallenblasen-Kontraktion beim Menschen durch Somatostatin. Dtsch Med Wochenschr 100:1135, 1975

33. Levin G, Malmud L, Rock E, et al: Effects of somatostatin on gallbladder emptying in man. Clin. Res. 31:284A, 1983

34. Boden G, Sivitz MC, Owen OE, et al: Somatostatin suppresses secretin and pancreatic exocrine secretion. Science 190:163, 1975

35. Schusdziarra V, Zyznar E, Rouiller D, et al: Splanchnic somatostatin: A hormonal regulator of nutrient homeostasis. Science 207:530, 1980

36. Bloom SR, Mortimer CH, Thorner MO, et al: Inhibition of gastrin and gastric-acid secretion by growth-hormone-release-inhibiting hormone. Lancet 2:1106, 1974

37. Mukai K, Greider MH, Grotting JC, et al: Retrospective study of 77 pancreatic endocrine tumors using the immunoperoxidase method. Am J Surg Pathol 6:387, 1982

38. Jensen RT, Gardner JD, Raufman JP, et al: Zollinger-Ellison Syndrome: Current concepts and management. Ann Int Med 98:59, 1983

39. Noe BD, Fletcher DJ, Spiess J: Evidence for the existence of a biosynthetic precursor for somatostatin. Diabetes 28:724, 1979

40. Samols E, Weir GC, Ramseur R, et al: Modulation of pancreatic somatostatin by adrenergic and cholinergic agonism and by hyper-and hypoglycemic sulfonamides. Metabolism 27:1219, 1978 (Suppl. 1)

41. Boden G, Baile CA, McLaughlin CL, et al: Effects of starvation and obesity on somatostatin, insulin and glucagon release from an isolated perfused organ system. Am J Physiol 241:E215, 1981

42. Sano T, Kagawa N, Hizawa K, et al: Demonstration of somatostatin production in medullary carcinoma of the thyroid. Jpn J Clin Oncol 10:221, 1980

43. Saito S, Saito H, Matsumura M, et al: Molecular heterogeneity and biological activity of immunoreactive somatostatin in medullary carcinoma of the thyroid. J Clin Endocrinol Metab 53:1117, 1981

44. Roos BA, Lindall AW, Ells J, et al: Increased plasma and tumor somatostatin-like immunoreactivity in medullary thyroid carinoma and small cell lung cancer. J Clin Endocrinol Metab 52:187, 1981

45. Ghose RR, Gupta SK: Oat cell carinoma of bronchus presenting with somatostatinoma syndrome. Thorax 36:550, 1981

46. Berelowitz M, Szabo M, Barowsky HW, et al: Somatostatin-like immunoactivity and biological activity is present in a human pheochromocytoma. J Clin Endocrinol Metab 56:134, 1983

47. Saito H, Saito S, Sano T, et al: Immunoreactive somatostatin in catecholamine-producing extra-adrenal paraganglioma. Cancer 50:565, 1982

# 5 | VIPoma Syndrome

*Thomas M. O'Dorisio*
*Hagop S. Mekhjian*

Shortly after the original description of the ulcerogenic syndrome,[1] it was noted that certain patients with nonbeta islet cell tumors and severe diarrhea did not meet the criteria for the diagnosis of gastrinoma. Verner and Morrison[2] and Priest and Alexander[3] were among the first to note the absence of gastric acid hypersecretion in such patients. In 1961 Murray, Paton, and Pope[4] documented achlorhydria in a patient presenting with this diarrhea non-beta cell pancreatic tumor syndrome. Matsumoto and colleagues termed the syndrome "pancreatic cholera" because the observed severe watery diarrhea resembled the clinical picture seen in Asiatic cholera.[5] In 1967, Marks, Bank and Louw proposed the acronym WDHA (*w*atery *d*iarrhea, *h*ypokalemia, *a*chlorhydria).[6] Since 1967, several studies have been reported confirming the association between certain pancreatic tumors and watery diarrhea syndrome. (WDS)[7-9]

## PATHOPHYSIOLOGY OF WDS

A brief review of the normal intestinal fluid transport seems relevant for the understanding of the pathophysiology of WDS. The normal intestinal tract receives about nine liters of fluid daily. This is comprised of salivary, gastric, pancreatic, biliary, and intestinal secretions. The maximal absorptive capacity of the small intestine is not known but is estimated to be about 12 liters. The small intestine absorbs most of this fluid load so that only one and one half liters reaches the ileocaecal valve.[10] The colon absorbs all but 100 ml of fluid which is excreted in the stool.[11] Perhaps more noteworthy is the fact that the colon can increase its absorptive capacity five- to six-fold, enabling it to absorb more than five liters of fluid per day.[12]

Normal absorption of fluid is the net effect of two distinct and somewhat independent processes. Absorption of fluid from lumen to plasma is a function of mature enterocytes at the villous tips, whereas secretion is thought to be a function of the crypt cells.[13] Any net increase of fluid volume in the intestinal tract could therefore result from a decrease in the absorption (or an increase) in the secretion of water. However, as long as the absorptive capacity of the colon is not exceeded there is no net change in fecal water loss. Diarrhea could be defined therefore, as a "malabsorption of water and electrolytes," clinically manifested by an increase in fecal weight.[14,15] There is no mechanism for the active absorption of water in the intestinal tract. Therefore, fluid absorption parallels the absorption and secretion of solutes.

Active and passive transport of ions occurs in the small and large intestine. There are significant regional differences in the relative contribution of active transport mechanisms to the overall fluid absorption in the intestinal tract. In the human jejunum, 85% of sodium and fluid absorption is accounted for by the passive movement of ions secondary to solvent drag (convection), created by the active absorption of nutrients such as amino acids and glucose.[16,17] Sodium-potassium activated ATP-ase, located at the basolateral membrane actively transports sodium into the intercellular space. The resulting fall in intracellular sodium concentration and the increase in potential difference favors sodium absorption along electrochemical gradients. In the presence of luminal bicarbonate, a sodium hydrogen exchange mechanism further enhances sodium absorption.[18] In addition to electrogenic sodium absorption, two ion exchange mechanisms account for most of the ion absorption in the ileum. Chloride-bicarbonate, and sodium-hydrogen exchange mechanisms result in neutral sodium chloride absorption.[19] Glucose contributes little, if any, to ileal sodium adsorption. The colon is quite similar to the ileum. Potassium transport is thought to be passive throughout the gastrointestinal tract, with the exception that potassium may be actively secreted in the colon.[20]

Active chloride secretion has been documented in the normal human jejunum[21] and guinea pig ileum.[22] A number of bacterial toxins, cholinergic agonists, and peptides, including VIP, have been demonstrated to produce active chloride secretion in vitro and bicarbonate secretion in vivo.[23] This secretion is thought to be mediated by an increase in cyclic AMP or alterations in intracellular calcium.[24,25]

A relatively small number of patients with WDS have been carefully studied with regard to alterations in intestinal absorptive function.[26-30] Three patients studied by Krejs et al. demonstrated a five-fold increase in the amount of endogenous fluid reaching the proximal jejunum. In addition, all three patients secreted sodium, chloride, and water in the jejunal test segment. Glucose absorption was lower than normal in these patients but the addition of glucose to the jejunal lumen stimulated sodium absorption. Although endogenous ileal flow was greatly increased, ileal absorption was normal or reduced and net ileal secretion could be demonstrated only when the concentration of the luminal sodium chloride was reduced to 5 mM. The latter observation suggests that the efficiency of ileal absorption is reduced in these patients.

The increased endogenous flow in the proximal intestine of these patients could be derived from secretion from the duodenum, the pancreas, or the hepatobiliary tree. In the patients studied by Modigliani et al.,[27,28] the endogenous flow at the ligament of Treitz was only slightly increased and the basal and stimulated pancreatic secretion was normal. In two of the patients studied by Soergel et al., the increased jejunal flow rate could only be demonstrated after a meal, suggesting an abnormal intestinal absorptive function and/or pancreatic response to a meal.[29] The dilute bile, high in the concentration of bicarbonate and chloride described in some patients[27] suggests, however, that biliary fluid secretion may play a role in the increased endogenous duodenal flow. The latter possibility is supported by the observation described in one patient in whom the entire diarrhea could be accounted for by massive pancreatic hypersecretion.[30]

Therefore, the diarrhea and the electrolyte abnormalities associated with the WDS are the result of: (1) increase in the endogenous flow at the ligament of Treitz, (2) marked increase in net jejunal water, sodium and chloride secretion; and (3) increased flow at the distal ileum associated with reduced ileal absorption. This set of events results in the daily delivery of 6.7–8.8 liters of fluid to the colon, overwhelming its absorptive capacity.[14] In addition VIP stimulated colonic secretion is likely to be present.[20] These result in large losses of bicarbonate in the stool.

The hypokalemia associated with WDS has been attributed to the loss of potassium from the gastrointestinal tract. Passive movements of potassium with bulk water flow in the small intestine and cyclic AMP mediated, active secretion of potassium by the large intestine[20] result in greater than 200 to 300 mEq of potassium losses in the stool. The colonic potassium loss is further aggravated by the secondary hyperaldosteronism associated with hypovolemia.[31] All of these findings provide a reasonable explanation for the metabolic hypokalemic hyperchloremic acidosis associated with WDS.

Hypochlorhydria is associated in 70% of patients with WDS.[32,33] Virtually all the peptides measured in plasma of patients with WDS are inhibitors of gastric acid secretion. In man VIP is a relatively weak inhibitor of pentagastrin stimulated gastric acid secretion,[34] which explains the absence of achlorhydria in many patients with WDS.

Flushing is seen in about 20% of patients with WDS.[33] This is presumed to be mediated by VIP which is a potent vasodilator in man.[35] A constant infusion of VIP produces a dose-dependent vasodilatation more pronounced in the region of the head. The vasodilatation disappears, however, in spite of the continued VIP infusions, presumably because of the development of tachyphylaxis.[36] The latter observation explains the occurrence of flushing only in 20% of patients with WDS. However, the possibility of a "surge" from a VIP producing tumor resulting in acute elevations with subsequent flushing cannot be excluded.

## THE ROLE OF VIP

Perhaps the single most important effect of VIP which has established it as the major modulator in WDS is its role as an intestinal secretagogue.

Its importance as both a normal neuromodulator of intestinal secretion and an abnormal "hormone" substance in WDS has been recently reviewed.[37,38]

Several important in vitro and, more recently, in vivo observations establishing VIP's mediating role in WDS will be briefly discussed. In 1974, Schwartz and colleagues reported that VIP produced net chloride secretion across rabbit and human ileal mucosa in vitro. The peptide increased short circuit current (in a dose-dependent manner) and produced chloride secretion in excess of sodium secretion.[39] Similar effects of VIP in the small intestine in vivo were noted in dog jejunal loops by Krejs and colleagues.[40] VIP infusion into superior mesenteric artery produced secretion of chlroide, potassium, bicarbonate, and water in dog jejunal loops. The magnitude of the secretion suggested that VIP produced active secretion of chloride and bicarbonate, creating a favorable gradient for the passive flux of potassium and perhaps sodium ions.[40] Essentially the same in vitro[39] and in vivo[40] effects of VIP on chloride secretion have been observed in man.[41] Krejs and Fordtran demonstrated in normal subjects that the human jejunum secreted chloride in response to increasing doses of VIP. The process was observed to be active, but the bicarbonate flux, unlike the canine model[40] remained unchanged.[41] Also noted in their study, the measured plasma VIP levels (by radioimmunoassay) achieved with the VIP infusion were in the order of magnitude observed in WDS, supporting the hypothesis that high levels of VIP could be responsible for certain secretory diarrheal states. Further, VIP has been observed to reverse the net chloride absorption to net secretion ratio in rat colon in vivo.[42] In these acute experiments, as well as others, [39-41] a high infusion dose of VIP was needed to cause chloride absorption to fall from a rate of 160 $\mu$Eq/10 min/g dry wt to secretion of 25 $\mu$Eq/10 min/g dry wt. This was accompanied by reversal of sodium and potassium absorption to secretion and a four fold increase of the existing bicarbonate secretion.[42]

The major problems with both in vitro and in vivo studies have been the short duration of study and the high VIP doses needed to effect intestinal secretion. Controversy in the literature revolved around whether or not VIP was only a marker for WDS and not in fact a causative agent.[43] Modlin and colleagues were one of the first groups to recognize that exogenous VIP administration for one or two hours (in pigs) did not mimic the condition in a patient with WDS who may be exposed to high concentrations of VIP for prolonged periods of time.[44] In their studies, infusion of VIP to achieve levels slightly above the upper range of normal (i.e. 180 pg/ml of plasma) induced cutaneous flushing and watery diarrhea. When VIP was infused chronically, six out of the eight pigs developed the flushing and watery diarrhea syndrome within ten hours of infusion. Most recently, VIP was given to normal subjects as a continuous intravenous infusion for 10 hours at a dose (400 pmol/kg/hr) which achieved RIA VIP levels within the range of those reported in patients with VIP secreting tumors.[45] All subjects developed profuse watery diarrhea in less than 6.5 hours. Stool analysis revealed the characteristics of secretory diarrhea, but no evidence of carbohydrate or fat malabsorption. There were also statistically significant increases in sodium and bicarbonate losses in the feces.[45]

This work, combined with studies demonstrating the presence of functional (i.e., stimulatable adenylate cyclase) VIP receptors on gut epithelial cells[46-48] has established not only the primary pathohumoral role of VIP in WDS but also alludes to its normal physiologic role as a local neuromodulator of intestinal secretion.[37,38] Although initially thought that intestinal motility in WDS was not enhanced, recent work suggests that intraarterially or intra-luminally administered VIP can indeed alter intestinal motor function, thus contributing to the diarrhea associated with WDS.[49]

In spite of the fact that VIP appears to be the leading candidate peptide for the modulation of WDS syndrome, there are some discrepancies that need explanation. VIP is thought to produce intestinal secretion by the stimulation of adenylate cyclase[50,51] and increase in cyclic AMP levels.[52] Where adenylate cyclase[53] and cyclic AMP levels[54,26] have been measured in patients with WDS syndrome, they have been found to be normal. The possibility exists that VIP produces intestinal secretion by a non-cyclic AMP mediated mechanism but, thus far, no such mechanism has been identified in patients with WDS. Conversely, it is possible that increases in cyclic AMP and adenylate cyclase may have been missed in measurements of whole mucosal biopsies. Because of intestinal cell heterogeneity, and the localization of adenylate cyclase and VIP receptors at the baso lateral membrane,[48] small changes in VIP responsive cell population could be missed. Other observations suggesting that VIP may not be the sole mediator of WDS include: the finding of normal VIP levels in some documented cases of WDS associated with hyperplasia of the pancreas; the response of the diarrhea to prostaglandin inhibitors such as indomethacin and, the presence of other elevated peptides with or without elevated VIP levels in some patients with WDS.[43,55] This latter possibility (that peptides other than VIP may play a role in WDS) is further supported by the relatively recent isolation of a 27 amino acid peptide, PHI (peptide histidine and isoleucine).[56,57] This peptide shares many sequence homologues with VIP, and some with secretin, glucagon, and GIP, indicating that it belongs to this family of peptides. Similar to VIP, PHI is found in the submucosa of the gut and is present in both brain and neural tissues, suggesting a neurotransmitter or neuromodulator role. Anagnastides and colleagues have recently infused PHI into normal volunteers.[58] In these studies PHI induced a secretion of chloride and sodium and either decreased net absorption or induced net secretion of water and potassium, while bicarbonate transport remained unaffected. Further, Bloom et al. have recenty reported the co-occurrence of PHI in 22 of 24 VIPomas.[59] At the present time, VIP must be considered to be the major mediator in WDS. Its augmenting secretory action with both PHI and other known and unknown peptides awaits further clarification.

## CLINICAL FEATURES

Episodic and often fulminating, secretory diarrhea in the WDS results in profound hypokalemia, hypochlorhydria (rarely achlorhydria), bicarbonate wasting, and hyperchloremic metabolic acidosis. The more commonly observed gastric hypochlorhydria is due to the direct gastric acid inhibitory effect of VIP, a biologic

**Table 5-1.** Effects of VIP Consistent with Signs and Symptoms of WDS

| Sign/Symptom | Incidence(%) |
|---|---|
| Secretory diarrhea | 100 |
| Hypokalemia (Mean K=2.2 mEq/L) | 100 |
| Hypochlorhydria | 70 |
| Hyperglycemia | 20–50 |
| Hypercalcemia | 25–75 |
| Flushing (vasodilation) | 20 |
| Atonic gallbladder | ? |

property shared with its other members of the secretin-glucagon family. As previously noted, the infrequent occurrence of pentagastrin stimulated achlorhydria in WDS is consistent with the properties of VIP as a relatively weak inhibitor of gastric secretion.[34] The incidence of signs and symptoms of WDS are shown in Table 5-1.[7,9,27,32,33,60,61] The most consistent clinical feature of the WDS entity associated with VIP tumors is the severe watery diarrhea and subsequent hypokalemia. In the early stage of tumor growth, the predominant symptoms of diarrhea are episodic and intermittent. It is generally accepted that, as the VIP tumor enlarges, the diarrhea becomes continuous and the ensuing electrolyte abnormalities life threatening.[7,9]

The hyperglycemia often noted in patients with WDS is probably secondary to the profound glycogenolytic effect of high portal vein VIP on the liver.[61] The observed hypercalcemia is poorly understood, but is also thought to be secondary to high VIP levels and enhanced osteolytic activity by VIP on the bone.[62] It should be noted, however, that this osteolytic activity on bone is not well documented. It may well be that a few VIPoma tumors are, indeed, part of the genetic multiple endocrine neoplasia syndrome (MEN-I) which includes parathyroid hyperplasia and hypercalcemia. Small vessel dilatation with secondary flushing and smooth muscle relaxation and atony of the small intestine have been well described and has already been alluded to.[7,9]

# DIAGNOSIS

The essential clinical criteria for the diagnosis of VIPomas are: (1) the establishment of the presence of secretory diarrhea; (2) identification of an intestinal secretagogue (VIP); and (3) the localization of the source of the production of the secretagogue.

The initial differentiation of secretory diarrhea from diarrhea of other causes can usually be made by some simple measurements. In secretory diarrhea the fecal water is greater than 500 ml and usually greater than 1 liter a day. The stool is isotonic with plasma and the sum of the concentration of stool sodium and potassium multiplied by two equals stool osmolality. Further, the diarrhea persists even after a 48–72 hour fast.

Once the diagnosis of chronic secretory diarrhea is established the differential diagnosis revolves around a limited number of other diseases associated with chronic secretory diarrhea. Most of these can usually be excluded by routine clinical and laboratory tests.[63,64] The major remaining diagnostic possibilities include the secretory diarrheas associated with peptide secreting tumors, chronic laxative abuse and "pseudopancreatic cholera."[64-66] An intestinal perfusion study demonstrating normal jejunal sodium and water absorption virtually rules out the diagnosis of pancreatic cholera. The differentiation of other chronic secretory diarrheas from VIPomas can only be made by normal plasma VIP levels (done in a reliable laboratory). This latter point is particularly important since a false positive value may subject the patient to exploratory surgery and unnecessary pancreatic restriction.

Table 5-2 contrasts WDS mediated by VIP secreting tumors with the Zollinger-Ellison syndrome. Differentiation of these two syndromes (see discussion of gastrinomas), in which diarrhea is often a dominant feature, cannot be made on clinical grounds alone; however, a few rather routine procedures and observations at the bedside can often differentiate between these two more common endocrine tumors. Nasogastric tube aspiration of acid and measurement of the aspirate pH will often alert the physician as to which line of tumor studies he should pursue. As can be noted in Table 5-2, measurement of stool pH, potassium, and bicarbonate (along with a review of the patient's serum electrolytes) is very useful and fairly easy to obtain in a hospital setting. The definitive diagnosis of the specific peptide secreting tumor associated diarrhea must rest on the measurement of the respective peptide in plasma.

Miscellaneous diagnostic procedures such as abdominal ultrasonography,[67] angiography,[68] and computerized axial tomography[69] are useful in the identification of sizable tumors of the pancreas. In cases of WDS associated with pancreatic hyperplasia these tests are usually negative. Furthermore these tests lack specificity and sensitivity.

**Table 5-2.** Differentiation of Zollinger-Ellison (ZES) and WDS (Verner-Morrison; WDHA)

| Feature | ZES | WDS |
|---|---|---|
| Diarrhea | Acid | Aklaline ($H_2CO_3$ loss) |
| Gastric acid | ↑↑↑ | ↓↓↓ |
| Gastric volume | ↑↑↑ | Normal |
| Nasal-gastric suction | ↓ Diarrhea | Diarrhea same |
| Motility | ↑↑* | → or slightly ↑ ** |
| Abdominal pain | +++ | Rare (initially) |
| Stool K$^+$ loss | Slightly ↑ | ↑↑↑ |
| Metabolic acidosis | No | Yes |
| Lesion-location | Pancreas | Pancreas (Adults) |
| | | Neuroblastomas (Children) |
| Mediator | Gastrin | VIP (primarily) |

* Motility enhanced secondary to acid succus from stomach.
** Motility may be slightly increased secondary to direct effects of either intra arterial or intra luminal VIP.[49]

## BIOCHEMICAL DIAGNOSIS AND EXPERIENCE

As alluded to above, biochemical detection of VIP secreting tumors necessitates a highly sensitive and specific VIP radioimmunoassay. We concur with the reported range of normal plasma VIP concentrations as being between 0 and 190 pg/ml.[62,70,71] Our reported range of normal VIP concentration for 100 fasting plasma samples is 0–170 pg/ml.[72]

It cannot be overemphasized that establishing the diagnosis of WDS due to a secreting tumor requires a thorough clinical evaluation and an elevated plasma VIP level. Information gained from a single plasma VIP level has only a limited usefulness to the physician who is forced into the difficult decision of submitting his patient to a surgical exploration. Further, it is possible that between periods of watery diarrhea, the VIPoma, not unlike many endocrine tumors of the gut (e.g., insulinoma, gastrinoma) may not be continuously secreting VIP; thus a "normal" level creates a false sense of security and may delay a more vigorous search for its cause.

Over the past four years, we have analyzed 2900 plasma samples for VIP sent to us from Canada and the United States with the suspected diagnosis of WDS. Of these, 29 patients were found to have elevated VIP levels in their plasma and later documented to have VIP secreting tumors at surgery. (Table 5-3) Our overall incidence of VIP-secreting tumors and WDS for all samples assayed was 1%. The mean age of our patients was $43 \pm 5$ years and the sex distribution was 11 males and 18 females. The normal mean plasma VIP for 100 normal fasting samples in our laboratory is $62 \pm 22$ (standard deviation) pg/ml with the range (already noted) of 0–170 pg/ml. The mean VIP values of our 29 documented VIP secreting tumors was $956 \pm 285$ (standard error) pg/ml. The standard deviation for this group of tumors was 457 pg/ml. The lowest initial VIP level in our 29 cases of VIPomas was 225 pg/ml (patient #16). This was from a sample drawn after the initial tumor was removed. This patient was found to have metastatic neuroblastoma with WDS. Our highest initial VIP value was 1850 pg/ml (patient #2, with metastatic ganglioneuroblastoma). Only four of 29 patients had VIPomas without metastasis at time of surgery, whereas 16 of 29 (56%) were found to have gross metastasis (usually to liver) at surgery. This finding compares with the series of Kraft and Colleagues[7] and probably reflects the rather long duration between symptoms and surgery (3 years), and the unavailability of reliable and clinically useful VIP RIAs.[7] Eight VIP-secreting ganglioneuroblastomas/phenochromocytoma tumors with WDS were noted in our series. Six of these eight (patients 2, 9, 15, 16, 18 and 20) were children less than five years of age. The other two patients (5 and 29) were adults and both had phenochromocytoma elements with their ganglioneuroblastoma tumors. Of interest, patient 13 had a documented small oat cell cancer of the lung associated with high VIP levels and the WDS, lending support to Said's original work which noted the association of VIP secreting tumors of the lung and the WDS.[71] Patient #25 is a patient with cutaneous mastocytoma and did not present as a classic WDS, but rather with flushing and hypotension. This patient has been recently reported.[73] Patient 14 was a 64-year-old woman with a VIP secreting tumor thought to arise from

**Table 5-3.** Documented VIP Secreting Tumors and WDS

| Patient | Age | Sex | VIP (pg/ml)* | Comment |
|---|---|---|---|---|
| 1 | 35 | M | 960 | Vipoma** |
| 2 | 2 | M | 1850 | Ganglioneuroblastoma** |
| 3 | 46 | M | 640 | Vipoma** |
| 4 | 40 | F | 1750 | Vipoma** |
| 5 | 53 | M | 880 | Pheo/ganglioneuroma |
| 6 | 62 | F | 1150 | Vipoma** |
| 7 | 36 | F | 280 | Vipoma** |
| 8 | 52 | M | 520 | Vipoma |
| 9 | 2 | F | 1700 | Ganglioneuroblastoma** |
| 10 | 38 | M | 1200 | Vipoma |
| 11 | 81 | F | 860 | Vipoma** |
| 12 | 70 | F | 320 | Vipoma** |
| 13 | 70 | M | 1500 | Small cell tumor of lung** |
| 14 | 64 | F | 540 | Vipoma** |
| 15 | 3 | F | 960 | Ganglioneuroblastoma |
| 16 | 3 | F | 225 | Neuroblastoma** |
| 17 | 48 | F | 640 | Vipoma** |
| 18 | 1 | F | 1000 | Ganglioneuroblastoma |
| 19 | 55 | F | 1250 | Vipoma** |
| 20 | 5 | F | 900 | Ganglioneuroblastoma |
| 21 | 50 | M | 1050 | Vipoma** |
| 22 | 50 | M | 850 | Vipoma** |
| 23 | 60 | F | 750 | Vipoma** |
| 24 | 50 | F | 1100 | Vipoma |
| 25 | 1 | F | 345 | Mast cell tumor+ |
| 26 | 75 | F | 1200 | Vipoma** |
| 27 | 68 | M | 880 | Vipoma** |
| 28 | 78 | M | 1800 | Vipoma** |
| 29 | 58 | F | 540 | Pheo/ganglioneuroblastoma |

* Normal mean = $62 \pm 22$ (Std Dev) pg/ml
** Indicates Metastasis
+ See Ref. 73. Symptoms in this patient were flush and syncope—not diarrhea.

the ovarian-uterine adnexa. In addition to elevated blood and tissue VIP levels (discussed below), she had elevated blood and tissue concentrations of somotostatin and neurotensin.

From our studies the incidence of false negative values which may have been present in the 2900 screened samples could not be determined. Attempts to gather this specific information and more detailed information on these patients have been, to date, unsuccessful. However, the overall mean VIP value of these 2900 samples (excluding the 29 surgically proven tumors) was 54 pg/ml, with 88% of these samples being below our limit of RIA detection (50 pg/ml plasma). This is in close agreement with the percent of samples that were below detection (90%) from the large screening study of Bloom and Polak.[9]

Pancreatic polypeptide (PP) was also screened in the plasma of the documented VIP-secreting tumor patients and was found to be elevated (i.e., >900 pg/ml) in 11 of 18 plasma samples studied. Although it is appealing to say that the high PP values marked probable localization of the VIP tumor to the pancreas, patients 5, 13, and 20 also had elevated plasma levels, but were found to have tumors of extrapancreatic origin.

Tissue VIP analysis on all the tumors listed has not been completed. However, we have some initial observations. Patients 2, 14, and 18 (ganglioneuroblastomas) had a mean VIP tumor level of 2.4 $\mu$g/g wet weight. Normal mean fresh adrenal (predominantly medulla) from 11 normal subjects is .012 $\pm$ .005 $\mu$g/g wet weight. No PP could be detected in any of these tumors. The mean VIP tumor concentration of patients 21 and 23 (both primary pancreatic and metastatic liver tumor) was 1.3 $\mu$g/g weight. Of interest, patients 21 and 23 had elevated fasting PP in their plasma (1050 and 2500 pg/ml respectively); however, the PP content in their tumors was not elevated (.030 and .016 $\mu$g/g wet weight; normal mean pancreatic PP concentrations being 0.034 $\mu$g/g, N = 4).

The above discussion and Table 5-3, out of necessity, represent only our initial observations on these 29 tumors. The acquisition of a complete profile of these patients and a more thorough analysis of the tumors has been painfully slow and in some instances precluded by the "lost to follow-up" notation from many of the physicians who have referred samples and information to our Center. However, we can appreciate that, when VIP is released from a tumor in high enough concentrations to exceed its peripheral degradating enzyme system, it behaves as a "hormone" in causing the WDS. Further, the possible co-occurrence of PHI and its significance needs to be evaluated.

## TREATMENT

The primary aim of the initial treatment is the replacement of fluid losses and correction of hypokalemia and acidosis. This could be attempted first, by the oral administration of glucose-electrolyte solutions. The advantage of oral over the intravenous route of supplementation is that orally administered glucose solutions enhance jejunal water and electrolyte transport, thereby reducing the net fluid loss from the gastrointestinal tract. Undoubtedly the magnitude and the route of fluid and electrolyte administration should be individualized and dictated by the severity of the deficits.

A number of pharmacologic agents that have been used in the control of the secretory diarrhea associated with VIPomas are listed in Table 5-4. These compounds work by either enhancing absorption or inhibiting intestinal secretion. The administration of the equivalent dose of 60–80 mg of Prednisone controls the diarrhea initially, in the majority of patients without any associated changes in plasma VIP levels.[74,75] The exact mechanism of the anti-diarrheal effect of Prednisone is not known. It is possible that in addition to the enhancement of sodium absorption in the jejunum[76] Prednisone alters the responsiveness of the intestinal "secretory apparatus" to the circulating secretagogue. Preliminary work in our laboratory using an acutely cell dispersed VIP-oma suggests that steroids produced a 40–50% inhibition of VIP release in vitro in a non dose dependent manner.

Among the pharmacologic agents that enhance sodium absorption, alpha adrenergic agonists,[77] angiotensin II and nor-epinephrine[78,79] have been shown to reduce the secretion associated with VIP secreting tumors or experimentally induced secretion by the exogenous administration of VIP.

**Table 5-4.** Therapy of WDHA Syndrome

I. Supportive
      Intravenous fluids
      Oral glucose electrolyte solutions
      Correct hypokalemia, acidosis
II. Pharmacotherapy
      Enhance absorption
         Corticosteroids
         Alpha 2 adrenergic agonists
         Angiotensin II
      Inhibit secretion
         Indomethacin
         Lithium carbonate
         Phenothiazines
         Somatostatin
         Opiates
         Propanolol
         Calcium channel blockers
         Adenylate cyclase inhibitors
III. Resection of Tumor
      Partial pancreatectomy
      "Debulking" of tumor
IV. Chemotherapy
      Streptozotocin
      5-Fluorofuracil
      Chlorozotocin

Indomethacin,[80,81] lithium carbonate,[82] somatostatin,[83-85] phenothiazines,[86,87] propanolol and other inhibitors of adenylate cyclase[88,89] have been used in the control of the secretory diarrhea associated with VIPomas. Phenothiazines compete with calcium for binding sites on the calcium binding protein, calmodulin, with resultant reduction of intracellular calcium and inhibition of secretion.[90] The mechanism of action of propanolol is not due to its beta blocking effect. It is possible that propanolol also influences the gating or mobilization of calcium in the intestinal cells and inhibits fluid secretion. It should be mentioned that, with the exception of steroids, none of these pharmacologic agents has been used consistently or in a sufficient number of patients with VIPomas to permit any strong conclusions about their therapeutic merit. They do, however, deserve further investigation.

The definitive treatment of VIPomas is surgery. Once the diagnosis is established, every patient should have an abdominal exploration. In the majority of instances the lesion is in the distal two thirds of the pancreas. Discrete tumors are reportedly found in 80% of patients. The literature claims that approximately 50% of VIPomas are benign and therefore potentially resectable. Further, islet cell hyperplasia or microadenomas are said to account for 20% of the well documented cases. A review of our experience with 29 cases (see Table 5-1) suggests that the majority of the patients have metastatic disease at the time of surgery. However, when a discrete tumor is identified it should be resected. Intra-operative ultrasonography has aided the identification of some small adenomas.[91] In the absence of a detectable pancreatic adenoma or other intraperitoneal tumors distal two third pancreatectomy is the surgical treatment of choice. A search for ganglioneuromas should also be carried out particularly in children since they account for 80% of the tumors associated with the WDS syndrome. For inoperable lesions, a "debulking" operation should be carried out with the hope of reducing the production of secretagogue and the tumor load for future chemotherapy. The postoperative course of some patients can be complicated by the occurrence of rebound gastric hypersecretion,[7,92,93] necessitating the use of $H_2$ receptor blockers. Postoperative fluid therapy can be complicated by the reversal of intestinal secretion and vasodilation and mobilization of large volumes of fluids.[94] For this reason careful monitoring of central venous pressures is mandatory in the management of these patients. Chemotherapy with streptozotocin and 5-FU[53,94] and more recently chlorozotocin is reported to give a 60–70% response rate, in some cases resulting in normalization of VIP levels and disappearance of diarrhea. Because of the episodic nature of the clinical manifestations of VIPomas, long periods of clinical remission can be expected.

# REFERENCES

1. Zollinger RM, Ellison EH: Primary peptic ulcerations of the jejunum associated with islet cell tumors of the pancreas. Ann Surg 142:709, 1955
2. Verner JV, Morrison AB: Islet cell tumor and a syndrome of refractory watery diarrhea and hypokalemia. Amer J Med 29:529, 1958
3. Priest WM, Alexander MK: Islet-cell tumor of the pancreas with peptic ulceration, diarrhea and hypokalemia. Lancet 2:1145, 1957
4. Murray JS, Paton RR, Pope CE II: Pancreatic tumor associated with flushing and diarrhea. Report of a case. N Engl J Med 264:436, 1961
5. Matsumoto KK, Peter JB, Schultze RG, et al: Watery diarrhea and hypokalemia associated with pancreatic islet cell adenoma. Gastroenterology 52:695, 1967
6. Marks IN, Bank S, Louw JH: Islet cell tumor of the pancreas with reversible watery diarrhea and achlorhydria. Gastroenterology 52:695, 1967
7. Kraft AR, Tompkins RK, Zollinger R: Recognition and management of the diarrheal syndrome caused by non-beta cell tumors of the pancreas. Am J Surg 119:163, 1970
8. Verner JV, Morrison AB: Endocrine pancreatic islet disease with diarrhea: Report of a case due to diffuse hyperplasia of non beta islet tissue with a review of 54 additional cases. Arch Intern Med 133:492, 1974
9. Bloom SR, Polak JM: Vipomas. In: Vasoactive Intestinal Peptides, p. 457, ed. Said SI. Raven Press, New York, 1982
10. Phillips SF, Giller J: The contribution of the colon to electrolyte and water conservation in man. J Lab Clin Med 81:733, 1973
11. Goy JAE, Eastwood MA, Mitchell WD, et al: Fecal characteristics contrasted in the irritable bowel syndrome and diverticular disease. Am J Clin Nutr 29:1480, 1976
12. Debongnie JC, Phillips SF: Capacity of the human colon to absorb fluid. Gastroenterology 74:698, 1978
13. Field M: Cholera toxin, adenylate cyclase, and the process of active secretion in the small intestine: The pathogenesis of diarrhea in cholera. In: Physiology of Membrane Disorders, p. 877, eds. Andreoli TE, Hoffman JE, Ianestil DD. Plenum Medical Book Company, New York, 1978
14. Fordtran JS: Speculations on the pathogenesis of diarrhea. Fed Proc 26:1405, 1967

15. Phillips SF: Diarrhea: A current view of pathophysiology. Gastroenterology 63:495, 1972
16. Fordtran JS: Stimulation of active and passive sodium absorption by sugars in the human jejunum. J Clin Invest 55:728, 1975
17. Fordtran JS, Rector Jr. FC, Carter NW: The mechanism of sodium absorption in the human small intestine. J Clin Invest 47:884, 1968
18. Turnberg LA, Fordtran JS, Carter NW, Rector FC: Mechanism of bicarbonate absorption and its relationship to sodium-transport in the human jejunum. J Clin Invest 49:548, 1970
19. Turnberg LA, Bieberdorf FA, Morawski SG et al.: Interrelationships of chloride, bicarbonate, sodium and hydrogen transport in the human ileum. J Clin Invest 49:557, 1970
20. Foster ES, Sandle GI, Hayslett JP, Binder HJ: Cyclic adenosine monophosphate stimulates active potassium secretion in the rat colon. Gastroenterology 84:324, 1983
21. Davis GR, Santa Ana CA, Morawski S, Fortran JS: Active chloride secretion in the normal human jejunum. J Clin Invest 66:1326, 1980
22. Powell DW, Binder HJ, Curran PF: Electrolyte secretion in the guinea pig ileum in vitro. Am J Physiol 223:531, 1972
23. Phillips SF, Gaginella TS: Intestinal secretion as a mechanism in diarrheal disease. In: Progress in Gastroenterology Vol II, p 481, ed. George BJ Glass. Grune & Stratton Inc., 1977
24. Field M: Intestinal Secretion. Gastroenterology 66:1063, 1974
25. Ilundain A, Naftalin RJ: Role of $Ca^{++}$ dependent regulator protein in intestinal secretion. Nature 279:446, 1979
26. Krejs GJ, Walsh JJ, Morawski BA, Fordtran JS: Intractable diarrhea: Intestinal perfusion studies and plasma VIP concentrations in patients with pancreatic cholera syndrome and Surreptitious Ingestion of laxatives and diuretics. Am J Digestive Diseases 22:280, 1977
27. Rambaud JR, Modiglianni R, Matuchansky S, et al: Pancreatic cholera. Studies on tumoral secretion and pathophysiology of diarrhea. Gastroenterology 69:110–122, 1975
28. Modiglianni R, Rambaud JC, Matuchansky C, Bernier JJ: Hormones intestinal secretion and diarrhea: human studies. In: Frontiers of the Knowledge of Diarrheal Disease, p. 289–302, eds. Janowitz HD, Sachar DB. Projects in Health Inc., NJ, 1979
29. Soergel KH, Bjork JT, Wood CM: The WDHA Syndrome: No correlation between clinical course, Plasma hormone levels and small intestinal function. In: Diarrhea in Disorders of Intestinal Transport, p. 133, eds. Rupper H, Domschke W, Soergel KH. Thieme Stratton Inc., New York, 1981
30. Schmitt MG, Soergel K, Hensley GT et al.: Watery diarrhea associated with pancreatic islet cell carcinoma. Gastroenterology 69:206, 1975
31. Levitan R, Ingelfinger FJ: Effect of d-aldosterone on salt and water absorption from the human colon. J Clin Invest 44:801, 1965
32. Verner JV, Morrisson AS: Non-B islet tumors and the syndrome of watery diarrhea, Hypokalemia and Hypochlorhydria. Clinics in Gastroenterology 3:595, 1974
33. Bloom SR, Long RG, Bryant MG, et al: Clinical, biochemical and pathological studies on 62 VIPomas. Gastroenterology 78:1143, 1980
34. Holm-Bentzen M, Schultz A, Fahrenkrug J, et al: Effect of VIP on gastric acid secretion in man. Hepatogastroenterology, 27 (Suppl.) 126, 1980
35. Domschke S, Domschke W, Bloom SR, et al: Vasoactive intestinal peptide in man: Pharmokinetics, metabolic and circulatory effects. Gut 19:1049, 1978
36. Modlin IM, Bloom SR, Mitchell SJ: Experimental evidence for vasoactive intestinal peptide as the cause of the watery diarrhea syndrome. Gastroenterology 75:1051, 1978

37. Gaginella TS, O'Dorisio TM: Vasoactive intestinal polypeptide: Neuromodulator of Intestinal Secretion on Mechanisms of Intestinal Secretion, p. 231–247, ed. Binder HJ, Alan R. Liss, Inc., New York, 1979
38. Gaginella TS, Hubel KA, O'Dorisio TM: Effects of Vasoactive Intestinal Peptide on Intestinal Chloride Secretion. Ibid ref. 9, 1982, p. 211–221
39. Schwartz CJ, Kimberg DV, Sheerin HE, et al: Vasoactive intestinal peptide stimulation of adenylate cyclase and active electrolyte secretion in intestinal mucosa. J Clin Invest 54:536, 1974
40. Krejs GJ, Barkey RM, Read NW, Fordtran JS: Intestinal secretion induced by vasoactive intestinal polypeptide. J Clin Invest 61:1337, 1978
41. Krejs GJ, Fordtran JS: Effect of VIP infusion on water and ion transport in the human jejunum. Gastroenterology 78:722, 1980
42. Wu, ZC, O'Dorisio TM, Cataland S, et al: Effects of pancreatic polypeptide and vasoactive intestinal polypeptide on rat ileal and colonic water and electrolyte transport in vivo. Dig Dis Sci 24:625, 1979
43. Gardner JD, McCarthy DM: VIP and watery diarrhea I—arguments against VIP being the cause of the watery diarrhea syndrome. In: Gut Hormones, pp. 570–573, ed. Bloom SR. Edinburgh, Churchill Livingstone, 1978
44. Modlin IM, Bloom SR, Mitchell SJ: Experimental evidence for vasoactive intestinal peptide as the cause of the watery diarrhea syndrome. Gastroenterology 75:1051, 1978
45. Kane MG, O'Dorisio TM, Krejs GJ: Intravenous VIP infusion causes secretory diarrhea in man. N Engl J Med 309:1482, 1983
46. Amiranaff B, Laburthe M, Rosselin G: Characterization of specific binding sites for vasoactive intestinal peptide in rat intestinal epithelial cell membrane. Biochem Biophys Acta 627:215, 1980
47. Binder HJ, Lemp GF, Gardner JD: Receptors for vasoactive intestinal peptide and secretion on small intestinal epithelial cells. Am J Physiol, GI-Liver Physiol I: G190, 1980
48. Dharmsathaphorn K, Harms V, Yamashiro DJ, et al: Preferential Binding of vasoactive intestinal polypeptide to basolateral membrane of rat and rabbit enterocytes. J Clin Invest 71:27, 1983
49. Snisky CA, Wolfe MM, Martin JL, et al: Effect of intravenous and intraluminal infusions of vasoactive intestinal peptide on myoelectric activity of rabbit small intestine. Am J Physiol 244 (7):G46, 1983
50. Simon B, Czygan P, Spaan G, et al: Hormone sensitive adenylate cyclase in human colonic mucosa. Digestion 17:229, 1978
51. Klaverman HL, Conlon TP, Levy AG, Gardner JD: Effects of gastrointestinal hormones on adenylate cyclase activity in human jejunal mucosa. Gastroenterology 68:667, 1975
52. Dupont C, Laburthe M, Broyart JP, et al: Cyclic AMP production in isolated colonic epithelial crypts: A highly sensitive model for the evaluation of vasoactive intestinal peptide action in human intestine. European J of Clin Invest 10:67–76, 1980
53. Kahn CR, Levy AG, Gardner JD, et al: Pancreatic Cholera: Beneficial effects of treatment with streptozotocin. N Engl J Med 292:941, 1975
54. Schwartz SE, Fitzgerald MA, Levine RA, Schwartzel EH: Normal jejunal cyclic nucleotide in a patient with secretory diarrhea. Arch Int Med 138:1403, 1978
55. Jaffe B: To be or not to VIP. Gastroenterology 76:417, 1979
56. Tatemoto K, Mutt V: Isolation of two novel candidate hormones using a chemical method for finding naturally occurring polypeptide. Nature 285:417, 1980
57. Tatemoto K, Mutt V: Isolation of the intestinal peptide porcine PHI (PHI 1–27), a new member of the Glucagon secretin family. Proc Nat Acad Sci 78:6603, 1981

58. Anagnastides AA, Christofides ND, Tatemoto K, et al: Peptide Histidine Isolencine (PHI): A new secretagogue in human intestine. Gut (In Press)

59. Bloom SR, Christofides ND, Yiangan T, et al: Peptide histidine isolencine (PHI) and Verner–Morrison Syndrome. Gut 24:473, 1983

60. Bloom S, Polak JM: Glucagonomas, VIPomas and somatostatinomas. Clinics in Endocrinology and Metabolism 9:285, 1980

61. Go VLW, Korinek JK: Effect of vasoactive intestinal polypeptide on hepatic glucose release. In: Vasoactive Intestinal Peptide. Ibid ref 9, 1982, p. 231

62. Bloom SR, Polak JM: VIP measurement in distinguishing Verner-Morrison syndrome and pseudo-Verner-Morrison syndrome. Clin Endocrin (Suppl) 5:223s, 1976

63. Matseche JW, Phillips SF: Chronic diarrhea. A practical approach. Med Clin N America 62:141, 1978

64. Morris AI, Turnberg LA: Surreptitious laxative abuse. Gastroenterology 77:780, 1979

65. Read NW, Read MG, Krejs GJ, et al: A report of five patients with large volume secretory diarrhea but no evidence of endocrine tumor or laxative abuse. Dig Dis Sci 27:193, 1982

66. Read WN, Krejs G, Read MG, et al: Chronic diarrhea of unknown origin. Gastroenterology 78:264, 1980

67. Shawker TH, Doppman JL, Dunnick NR, et al: Ultrasonic investigation of pancreatic islet cell tumors. J Ultrasound Med 1:193, 1982

68. Gold RP, Black TJ, Rotterdan H, Casarella WJ: Radiologic and pathologic characteristics of the WDHA syndrome. Am J Roentegenol 127:397, 1976

69. Moss AA: Computed axial tomographic scanning, In: Gastrointestinal Disease. Pathophysiology, diagnosis, management. Slesinger and Fordtran (eds), WB Saunders Co., 1983, p. 1707

70. Ebeid AM, Murray PD, Fisher JE: Vasoactive intestinal peptide and the watery diarrhea syndrome. Ann Surg 187:411, 1978

71. Said SI, Faloona GR: Elevated plasma and tissue levels of vasoactive intestinal polypeptide in the watery-diarrhea syndrome due to pancreatic, bronchogenic and other tumors. N Engl J Med 293:155, 1975

72. O'Dorisio TM: VIP and watery diarrhea. In: Gut Hormones (ed. S. R. Bloom), Edinburgh, Churchill-Livingstone, 1978, p. 581

73. Wesley RR, Vinik AI, O'Dorisio TM, et al: A new syndrome of symptomatic cutaneous mastocytoma producing vasoactive polypeptide (VIP). Gastroenterology 80:963, 1982

74. Barraclough MA, Bloom SR: VIPoma of the Pancreas. Observations on the diarrhea and circulatory disturbances. Arch Int Med 139:467, 1969

75. Lennon JR, Sircus W, Bloom SR, et al: Investigation and treatment of recurrent VIPoma. Gut 16:821, 1975

76. Charney AN, Donowitz M: Prevention and reversal of cholera enterotoxin-induced intestinal secretion by methyl prednisolone induction of Na+ − K+ − ATPase. J Clin Invest 57:1590, 1976

77. McArthur KE, Anderson SD, Durbin TE, et al: Clondine and Lidamidine to inhibit watery diarrhea in a patient with lung cancer. Ann Int Med 96:323, 1982

78. Rao MB, O'Dorisio TM, George JM, et al: Angiotensin II and nor-epinehrine antagonize the effect of vasoactive intestinal peptide on rat ileum and colon. Peptides (In Press)

79. Field M, McColl I: Ion transport in rabbit ileal mucosa III. Effects of cathcolamines. Am J Physiol 225:852, 1973

80. Jaffe BM, Kopen DF, DeSchryver-KecsKemeti K, et al: Indomethacin-responsive pancreatic cholera. New England J Med 297:817, 1977

81. Albuquerque RH, Owens CWI, Bloom SR: A study of vasoactive intestinal polypeptide

(VIP) stimulated intestinal fluid secretion in rat and its inhibition by indomethacin. Experientia 35:1496, 1979

82. Pandol SJ, Korman LY, McCarthy DM, Gardner JD: Beneficial effects of oral lithium carbonate in the treatment of pancreatic cholera syndrome. New Eng J Med 302:1403, 1980

83. Dharmsathaphorn K, Sherwin RS, Dobbins JW: Somatostatin inhibits fluid secretion in the rat jejunum. Gastroenterology 78:1554, 1980

84. Dharmsathaphorn K, Binder JJ, Dobbins JW: Somatostatin stimulates sodium and chloride absorption in the rabbit ileum. Gastroenterology 78:1559, 1980

85. Carter RE, Bitar KN, Zfass AM, Makhlouf GM: Inhibition of VIP stimulated intestinal secretion and cyclic AMP production by somatostatin in the rat. Gastroenterology 74:726, 1978

86. Donowitz M, Elta G, Bloom SR, Nathanson L: Trifluoroperazine reversal of secretory diarrhea in pancreatic cholera. Ann Int Med 93:284, 1980

87. Smith PL, Field M: In vitro antisecretory effects of trifluoroperazine and other neuroleptics in rabbit and human small intestine. Gastroenterology 78:1545, 1980

88. Waldman DB, Gardner TD, Zfass AM, Makhlouf GM: Effects of vasoactive intestinal peptide, secretin, and related peptides on rat colonic transport and adenylate cyclase activity. Gastroenterology 73:518, 1977

89. Makhlouf G: Adenylate cyclase inhibitors. In: Frontiers of Knowledge in the Diarrheal Diseases, edited by HD Janowitz and DB Sachar. Projects in Health Inc., Upper Montclair, NJ, 1979, p. 337

90. Klee CB, Crouch TH, Richman PG: Calmodulin. Ann Rev Biochem 49:489, 1980

91. Charboneau JW, James EM, Van Herden JA, et al: Intraoperative real time ultra sonographic localization of pancreatic insulinoma: Initial Experience. J Ultrasound Med 2:251, 1983

92. Sansenbacher LJ, Mekhjian HS, King DR, et al: Studies on the potential role of secretin in the islet cell diarrheogenic syndrome. Ann Surg 119:163, 1970

93. Anderson H, Detevall G, Fagerberg G, et al: Pancreatic tumor with diarrhea, hypokalemia and hypochlorhydria. Acta Chir Scand 138:102, 1972

94. Moertel CG, Hanley JA, Johnson LA: Streptozotocin alone compared with streptozotocin plus fluorouracil in the treatment of advanced islet-cell carcinoma. N Engl J Med 303:1189, 1980

# 6 Pancreatic Polypeptide- and Mixed Peptide- Producing Tumors of the Gastrointestinal Tract

*Thomas M. O'Dorisio*
*Aaron I. Vinik*

The past decade has witnessed and monitored the rapidly growing field called gastrointestinal (GI) endocrinology.[1] Advances in biochemical peptide purification and the development of both highly specific radioimmunoassay and immunocytochemistry have created a rich and fertile milieu for basic and clinical investigations.[2] For the clinician, the greatest area of interest lies in information generated on peptide-producing tumors of the GI tract.[3-7] The intent of this chapter is to establish a practical understanding of the GI endocrine cell system and to relate this system to functioning (defined clinical syndromes) and nonfunctioning (without defined clinical syndromes) endocrine tumors of the gut.

## THE GI ENDOCRINE CELL/TUMOR SYSTEM: PRACTICAL GUIDELINES

Although detailed discussion of the GI endocrine cell has been included in this book (Chapter 1), certain concepts and guidelines should be delineated. They are needed to better understand the pathophysiologic behavior of GI endocrine tumors.

117

GI endocrine cells elaborate polypeptide substances (in many cases, hormones) and not substances composed of thyronines or sterols (e.g., thyroxine and glucocortocoids).[8] Synthesis of these latter molecules requires several specialized enzymes not present in the GI endocrine cell. By contrast, the GI endocrine cell can effect polypeptide biosynthesis with fewer, less specialized enzymes and cytoplasmic ribonucleic acids already in place for synthesis of other cell proteins.[8] It should also be recognized that the vast majority of GI peptides thus far isolated and/or identified with specific endocrine cells of the GI tract are candidate hormones only and have not as yet met accepted physiologic criteria of a gastrointestinal hormone as proposed by Grossman (Table 6-1).[9] To date, only four of the many chemically defined peptides extracted from the GI tract have achieved classic hormone status; namely, gastrin, cholecystokinin (CCK), secretin, and gastric inhibitory peptide (GIP). The physiologic aspects of these hormones and other GI peptides are reviewed elsewhere. To date, the only GI hormone clearly established in a pathophysiologic tumor state is gastrin (gastrinoma, Zollinger-Ellison syndrome). Secretin and CCK secreting tumors have not been reported. A GIP secreting tumor was reported, but subsequently retracted. Gastrinoma, insulinoma, and glucagonoma constitute the only tumors of the entero-pancreatic system which secrete true hormones. The pathophysiologic features of these tumors could be predicted from their known physiologic effects. By contrast, such peptides as vasoactive intestinal peptide (VIP, vipoma) somatostatin (somatostatinoma), and pancreatic polypeptide (PP, PPoma) are "hormones" only in the pathophysiological sense and the normal physiologic function extrapolated from observations of their oversecretion. Frequently observed co-occurrence of these peptides with gastrinoma, insulinoma, and glucagonoma (discussed below) aids us in developing general concepts and a practical understanding not only regarding the GI endocrine cell system, but the enteropancreatic tumor system as well. Since certain neurogenic tumors (i.e., pheochromocytoma, neuroblastoma) contain several GI peptides including somatostatin, VIP and enkephlin[10-12] and, because many of the GI peptides occur both in their respective endocrine cells as well as in nerves (e.g., VIP, somatostatin, gastrin, and CCK), we need to recognize that "endocrine" tumors of the enteropancreatic system may be either of endocrine or neurocrine origin. The gastrointestinal enteropancreatic axis embraces both endocrine and neurocrine tumors.

Although controversy exists regarding both the exact site of origin of the GI endocrine cell and the etiology of the endocrine tumor secreting cell, the hypothesis of A.G.E. Pearse is appealing. Pearse drew from the observations of the German

**Table 6-1.** Criteria for a Gastrointestinal Hormone

1. Physiologic stimulus effects release of endocrine cell substance in the G.I. tract.
2. This substance effects response on a distant organ.
3. Extraction of that part of the G.I. tract to which the stimulus is applied effects a similar response.
4. Effect on target organ can be mimicked by exogenous infusion of this substance in amounts and identical molecular form that copy the observed endogenous release following the physiologic stimulus(i).

Modified from Grossman MI: Physiological effects of gastrointestinal hormones. Fed Proc 36:1930, 1977 morphologist, Feyrter, that the "clear cells" of the GI tract possessed the special property of reducing silver salt (argentaffin) or could at least take up silver salts, which could subsequently be reduced (argyrophil).[13] In 1966, Pearse put forth the unifying hypothesis that all peptide-producing cells of both gut and pancreas belong to a much larger group of cells having many common cytochemical, ultra-structural, and functional characteristics.[14] The acronym APUD was invented to reflect the *a*mine *p*recursor *u*ptake *d*ecarboxylation characteristics of these tumors. According to Pearse and colleagues, the cells and their respective APUD-omas are thought to derive from neuro or specialized ectoderm, but not from the entoderm of the gut wherein they have come to reside.[15] Weichert supported Pearse's concept and expanded the theory.[16] He proposed that certain polypeptide-producing cells of the pancreas, thyroid, lung, parathyroid, adrenal, and GI mucosa are derived from neuroectodermal cells, which migrate into the primitive alimentary mucosa and are passively carried (during organ differentiation) to their definitive position where they mature.[16]

Several investigators, using quail chicken chimera and labelled cell-chase histochemical and electromicroscopic methodology, could not fully support the neuroectodermal derivation of the GI endocrine cell.[17-19] At the present time, the exact tissue origin of the GI endocrine system is not resolved. However, on a more practical basis, the APUD concept provides a convenient framework with which to address another important postulate regarding the endocrine cell system; namely, the toti-potential nature and multi-peptide producing ability of these cells.[8] Drawing from the work of several investigators,[20-22] Omen hypothesized "depression" of genetic structural information as a unifying mechanism for relating the observed neoplastic transformation of a cell and its production of a polypeptide substance (e.g., gastrin hormone) to a general biological principle of control. Support of this single toti-potential cell proposal has come from Creutzfeldt and colleagues. They have reported work that suggests the $D_1$ cell (normally present in the pancreatic islet of Langerhans) is a precursor or "stem-cell" capable of both differentiating into matrix endocrine cells and also of producing a variety of other peptides.[23] Although Omen's theory leaves unanswered why or how genes are "derepressed" it does not help us to understand the co-occurrence of multiple endocrine neoplasia (MEN) with such endocrine tumors as gastrinoma and insulinoma (discussed below).

If we accept, for the purposes of discussion, that the APUD cells and their respective tumors are of a toti-potential nature, capable of both genetic or acquired(?) gene-derepression, then several general observations regarding multiple peptide (often hormone) production by a single tumor can be made. Endocrine tumors of the gut may produce orthocrine peptides (i.e., their natural product); examples include insulinoma, glucagonoma, and gastrinoma. Further, they may produce foreign peptides as well either from different peptide-secreting cells within the tumor or by the same cell synthesizing more than one substance.

A plausible explanation for multiple hormone production is the tumor synthesis of a common ancestral peptide which is variably processed in the different tissues. Thus, the possibilities for explaining multiple hormone production by mixed pancreatic tumors are many and include: (1) a single-cell type with single precursor molecule; (2) a single-cell type with a common precursor molecule; (3) a single-cell type and a separate precursor molecule; (4) multiple-cell types with multiple molecules; and (5) multiple cell types but a single peptide-secreting clone.[15] The peptides thus released from an endocrine tumor may mediate release of another peptide(s) from the same or distant organ (i.e., in a paracrine or endocrine manner), and functioning pancreatic tumors (e.g., gastrinoma) with multiple endocrine neoplasia syndrome and its respective hypersecreting endocrine gland(s) also associated with multiple peptide secretion can occur.

Clinically, the vast majority of patients with mixed pancreatic endocrine tumors present with symptoms characteristic of secretion of only *one* peptide. In some cases (gastrinoma, glucogonoma, insulinoma), the predominating peptide is a hormone and its physiologic and pathologic behavior well known and relatively easy to diagnose. It is the so-called nonfunctional endocrine tumors which may secrete several peptides whose physiologic and pathophysiologic function is less well defined that will be most troublesome to the clinician trying to make a diagnosis. An example of a peptide seeking a physiological function and commonly associated with GI enteropancreatic tumors is pancreatic polypeptide (PP, discussed below).

## PANCREATIC POLYPEPTIDE (PP) AND THE ENDOCRINE TUMORS OF THE ENTEROPANCREATIC SYSTEM

Oversecretion of PP is one of the most frequent associations noted with well defined functioning endocrine tumors.[3,23-27] This polypeptide was independently isolated and characterized by both Chance and colleagues[28] and Kimmel and associates.[29] In man, PP is localized almost exclusively (93%) to the secretory granules of a distinct endocrine cell type in the pancreas. These cells are located predominantly in the head of the pancreas (both within the islets and scattered about the exocrine parenchyma). The exact physiologic function of PP in man is not known. Stimulation of its release is, however, nutrient-, cerebro-, and hormone (CCK, secretin)-mediated. Recent work in man suggests that PP is an inhibitor of both pancreatic enzyme secretion and bile acid output in physiologic concentrations.[30] However, these functions are not regularly detected clinically.

In their early work, Polak and colleagues suggested that PP may serve as a general marker for several endocrine tumors of the pancreas.[24] Other studies have confirmed the co-occurrence of elevated PP concentrations in either blood or extracts of tumor tissue in functioning endocrine tumors of the pancreas.[31-32] It now appears that PP cells can be involved in endocrine tumors of the pancreas: as a "pure" PP cell tumor; in mixed endocrine tumors or; as PP cell hyperplasia in extratumoral pancreatic tissue (i.e., pancreatic tissue not involved with the tumor).

Endocrine tumors consisting predominantly of PP cells are clinically silent. As a result, the presenting clinical symptoms may be only of the tumor mass.[3] Table 6-2 summarizes the frequency of elevated PP (either in tumor or in blood), collated from several series.[3,23-27] Frequent occurrence of this peptide in the func-

**Table 6-2.** Frequency of PP-Containing Cells in the Major Functioning Enteropancreatic Endocrine Tumors

| Tumor | Percent of PP increased[a] | |
|---|---|---|
| | Basal Blood (>900 pg/ml) | Tissue (cells) |
| Gastrinoma | 26 | 18 |
| Insulinoma | 22 | 33 |
| Vipoma | 71[b] | 58[c] |
| Glucagonoma | 50 | 44[d] |
| Carcinoid | 29 | 30?[e] |

[a] Mean percent gathered from several studies[3,23-27]
[b] Includes frequency of PP elevation in our VIPoma series (Chapter 5)
[c] Includes both detectable PP cells and/or elevated concentrations measured in tissue extract by RIA.
[d] Range on the small series of these tumors is 0–64%.
[e] From work of Solcia.[32]

tioning tumors gastrinoma, insulinoma, vipoma, glucagonoma, and carcinoid serves to point out an important aspect of multiple peptide secreting tumors. From Table 6-2, it can be seen that an excess of PP secretion is associated with tumors characterized by overproduction of a single substance (gastrin, insulin, VIP, glucagon, and serotonin) causing the clinical syndrome.

It has been suggested that raised plasma PP concentrations might be considered a useful marker in localizing endocrine tumors to the pancreas.[24] Further, elevated plasma PP may arise not only from PP cells found within certain functioning endocrine tumors but as hyperplastic PP cells in extratumoral pancreatic tissue; behaving in a "reactionary" manner to either the major peptide secreted by the tumor (in many instances, VIP) or a non-specific reaction of pancreatic tissue to injury.[26] This latter point is not obvious in Table 6-2, since the actual number of PP secreting cells in any of the given functioning tumor series is not shown. There does not appear to be a relationship between the number of PP cells and their function, since islet tumors containing subnormal, normal, or supranormal concentrations of PP (when compared with normal pancreas) may be associated with normal or high levels of circulating PP.[33] Recent studies suggest that raised PP concentrations occur with nonpancreatic endocrine tumors such as carcinoid. Elevated plasma PP is observed even when the carcinoid is isolated and outside the pancreas (Table 6-2).[3] This response may be due to stimulation of PP cells from humors elaborated by the extrapancreatic or carcinoid tumor.[3] A brief case serves to emphasize the difficulty in assessing the value of a high PP plasma level in association with a functioning endocrine tumor.

The patient is a 58-year-old woman who presented with severe watery diarrhea, hypokalemia, muscle weakness, and hypochlorhydria in response to pentagastrin stimulation. Fasting plasma PP values ranged between 700 and 900 pg/ml (normal <150 pg/ml), and VIP levels between 400 and 600 pg/ml (normal <50 pg/ml). A CT scan localized a left suprarenal mass. Work-up for pheochromocytoma was negative. At operation, no A-V gradient for PP or for VIP across the large suprarenal mass could be demonstrated. After removal of the ganglioneuroblastoma, plasma VIP, and PP returned to normal basal levels. VIP concentrations in the tumor extract was 960 ng per gram wet weight (normal adrenal medulla VIP is ≤18 ng/g wet weight), and there was no detectable PP in the tumor. The pancreas was not biopsied at the time of surgery; however, no detectable lesions were noted. The return of PP to normal after removal of VIP-secreting tumor implied that VIP may have exerted a "humoral" effect on normal pancreatic PP cells.

It is not clear whether or not non-endocrine tumors of the pancreas (e.g., adenocarcinoma) are associated with elevated blood or tissue PP concentrations. If cases were to be described, these would tend to support a release of PP from normal pancreatic tissue as a response to pancreatic injury.

Before leaving the discussion on the significance of PP elevation in endocrine tumors, another point already alluded to should be stressed: namely, many of the so-called "non-functional" endocrine tumors of the pancreas may well be principally PP-secreting tumors. Between 20 and 70% of these non-functional endocrine tumors have raised basal PP.[3,25,34] It should be kept in mind that elevation of PP occurs with advancing age, renal and liver disease, and in some unexplained cases of diarrhea. It may also be found in family members of MEN patients. Thus, the diagnosis of a PP-secreting tumor may prove difficult. A provocative secretin challenge, showing an exaggerated PP response in these patients as contrasted with a normal group may enhance the detection rate of these tumors.[3] Schwartz has suggested that administration of atropine will suppress PP concentrations in healthy subjects, but fails to do so in patients with pancreatic endocrine tumors.[35] This has not been examined in any large series. Clearly, more studies using provocative testing for PP release in a suspected state of an endocrine tumor are needed.

Nonetheless, an elevated basal PP of >1000 pg/ml in the absence of factors known to cause marked elevation of PP release (see above) may be an indication of a non-functioning pancreatic endocrine tumor. Non-invasive studies such as ultrasound and CT should always be done first, followed by angiography. These tumors are always highly vascular. Localization procedures which would include percutaneous transhepatic portal venous sampling looking for a clear gradient should be contemplated.[3] Finally, if there is evidence of PP overproduction (i.e., a step-up) across the pancreas, an exploratory laporatomy should be considered.

## MIXED PEPTIDE-PRODUCING TUMORS

We have reviewed the very frequent occurrence of PP with functioning endocrine tumors of the pancreas. With improved immunocytochemistry and specific peptide radioimmunoassay development, it has become apparent that mixed endocrine tumors of the pancreas are much more common than originally postulated. The mechanisms for multiple hormone production by a single tumor and, rarely, a single tumor cell, can again be better understood in light of the previously developed concepts of the GI endocrine system. It is neither surprising nor unexpected to see more than one peptide co-occurring with well-described pancreatic endocrine tumors. Table 6-3 demonstrates the frequency of mixed peptide production in

**Table 6-3.** Frequency of Mixed Peptide (Hormonal) Production in the Major Tumors of the Enteropancreatic System (% Increased)[a]

| Peptide | Gastrinoma | Insulinoma | Glucagonoma | Carcinoid[b] |
|---|---|---|---|---|
| Gastrin | 100 | 8 | 0 | 50 |
| Insulin | 29 | 100 | 50 | — |
| Glucagon | 20 | 20 | 100 | — |
| Somatostatin | 20 | 0 | 66 | 25 |
| ACTH/CLIP[c] | 30 | 11 | — | d |

[a] Mean percent increased from several series.[3,4,25-25,27,32]
[b] Data summarized from Reference 4.
[c] CLIP is Fragments 18–39 ACTH.
[d] Reported to be present, Reference 32.

tumors of the entero-pancreatic system. The mean percents are given in Table 6-3.[3,4,23-25,27,32] The production of almost all of the peptides listed in Table 6-3 have been reported in any one of the functional tumors. In general, most endocrine tumors are composed of several distinct endocrine cell types, with separate cells responsible for each peptide released.[25] We have noted earlier, that the peptide most frequently found in association with other pancreatic endocrine tumors is PP (cf, Table 6-2). An interesting parallel to the PP observation, but not reported in Table 6-3 is the study by Pearse and colleagues who examined non-tumor parts of the pancreas for somatostatin concentrations.[36] In 20 cases investigated, the number of somatostatin cells were increased fivefold in the uninvolved parts of the pancreas that contained a functioning pancreatic endocrine tumor (gastrinoma, insulinoma, glucagonoma, or vipoma). The most striking increase in somatostatin was found in the normal pancreas juxtaposed to VIP-producing tumors.[36] The increase of somatostatin may be similar to that found with PP and represents a pancreatic reaction to the presence of the tumor.[25] This may well be due in part to stimulation of the somatostatin or PP cells by the local excess of the peptide (e.g., gastrin, insulin, glucagon, or VIP) acting in a paracrine manner. At present, the significance of this extratumoral somatostatin and PP cell hyperplasia is not known.

Another observation from Table 6-3 bears mentioning; that is, the multiple peptide-secreting capacity of carcinoid tumors.[4,32] In addition to gastrin, somatostatin, and ACTH/CLIP (Fragment 18–39 of ACTH), substance P and motilin have also been localized to these tumors.[37,38] Carcinoid tumors have been recognized clinically and histologically longer than any of the other peptide-producing tumors of the GI tract.[39] They probably represent best the amine/peptide secreting cell of the gut APUD-oma series. Furthermore, carcinoids serve to interface MEN syndrome with endocrine APUD-omas.[40-43]

## MULTIPLE ENDOCRINE NEOPLASIA AND THE ENTEROPANCREATIC TUMORS

In the instance of carcinoid tumor and the associated MEN II (i.e., medullary thyroid carcinoma, parathyroid hyperplasia, and pheochromocytoma) we see an example of initial gene mutation[8] (thought to be an autosomal dominant pattern) affecting multiple clones of APUD cells (i.e., calcitonin-secreting cells of the thyroid, chief cells of the parathyroid, adrenal medullary cells, and often the enterochromoffin cells of the GI tract). These cells are diffusely distributed and result in various stages of hyperplasia (parathyroid gland), neoplasia (medullary thyroid carcinoma) or, often, cardinoid tumors.[41]

It is this association of carcinoid with Type II MEN and the greater than 80% occurrence of pancreatic APUD-omas in MEN Type I (pituitary adenoma and parathyroid hyperplasia),[42] that should alert the clinician to the important ramifications of this observation when pursuing a diagnostic evaluation in a patient with a possible endocrine tumor of the gut. Further, the classification of MEN I and II, particularly as they pertain to gut endocrine tumors may be arbitrary. In a recent study of 40 patients followed for 30 years, Zollinger and colleagues reported that 13 of 40 patients were classified as MEN I. Three of these 13 MEN I patients developed bilateral pheochromocytoma (not previously reported to be associated with MEN I) in the course of their 30 year follow-up. One of these patients had both a paraganglioneuroma and bilateral pheochromocytoma.[12] Preliminary work (University of Michigan, A.I. Vinik) using immunohistochemical techniques on 14 MEN I pancreatic tumors has identified the occurrence of both serotonin (4 of 14) and somatostatin (12 of 14) within the pancreatic tumors. Both serotonin (in the setting of carcinoid) and somatostatin (in medullary thyroid carcinoma tissue) occur in MEN II.[40,41] Although medullary thyroid carcinoma (associated with MEN II) has not been reported in an MEN I patient, calcitonin-secreting tumors have been reported in the gastrinoma of MEN I patients and in carcinoid tumors, the latter tumors associated with both MEN I and MEN II kindreds.[41,43] For the clinician, the ramifications of these observations are that the gut endocrine tumors are not only mixed and able to hypersecrete several peptides, but may also form part of an MEN syndrome which necessitates appropriate screening of several endocrine glands (including the adrenal medulla). This is especially important in patients with peptide ulcer disease, in whom raised gastrin levels may suggest a gastrinoma, but in whom the raised levels may, in fact, derive from

**Table 6-4.** Multiple Endocrine Neoplasia (MEN) and the Enteropancreatic Tumors

| Organ/Tumor | MEN I | MEN II |
|---|---|---|
| Pituitary | Yes[a] | No |
| Parathyroid | Yes[a] | Yes[d] |
| Pancreatic Tumor | Yes[a,b] | No |
| Pheochromocytoma | Yes[c] | Yes[d] |
| Medullary Thyroid Carcinoma | No | Yes[d] |
| Adrenal Cortex | Yes | Yes |
| Carcinoid | Yes | Yes |
| Neurofibromas/Lipomas | Yes | Yes |

[a] Major organ involvement for MEN I diagnosis[42]

[b] Pancreatic Tumors are mostly gastrinoma and insulinoma

[c] Recently described with MEN I/gastrinoma patients[12]

[d] Major organ involvement for MEN II diagnosis[43]

# 7 | Chemotherapeutic Management of Endocrine-Producing Tumors of the Gastrointestinal Tract

*Daniel G. Haller*

## INTRODUCTION

The relative rarity of endocrine-producing tumors of the gastrointestinal tract has made clinical investigations into the management of these malignancies extraordinarily difficult. Although the first chemotherapeutic treatment of a carcinoid tumor was reported over 25 years ago,[1] data supporting the optimal therapy of such patients have largely been anecdotal. In addition to the paucity of cases of islet cell malignancies and carcinoid tumors, other reasons help to explain the difficulties involved in the research for appropriate cytotoxic chemotherapy of these diseases:

1. The standard definitions of "benign" and "malignant" are often inappropriate when discussing the clinical course of these tumors. For many patients, the histologic diagnosis of a malignant carcinoid neoplasm may not adequately describe the indolent course characteristic of these tumors.

2. The availability of non-cytotoxic therapies for these patients may render patients relatively asymptomatic until very late in the course of their disease when

the introduction of aggressive chemotherapy may be difficult, if not impossible. Declining performance status, poor cardiac or renal function, and inadequate nutrition characteristic of end-stage disease in these patients may make the most effective known agents contraindicated. The timing of chemotherapy, therefore, represents a difficult clinical decision.

3. Although criteria of response have been well described for most tumors, the variable nature of endocrine tumors of the gastrointestinal tract has required more specific measurements relating not only to tumor size and patient survival, but also to hormone production and symptomatic or subjective improvement.

In spite of these problems, individual observations over the past quarter century have led to large multi-institutional studies which are providing guidelines for the more rational therapy of patients with functioning and non-functioning endocrine tumors of the gastrointestinal tract.

## CARCINOID TUMORS

The earliest report describing the use of cytoxic chemotherapy of a non-functioning carcinoid tumor appeared in 1957.[1] The patient presented initially in 1942 with a presumed adenocarcinoma of the rectum and was treated with surgery and post-operative radiation therapy. Six years later, liver metastases appeared and, because of symptomatic hepatomegaly, intraarterial nitrogen mustard was administered. A significant decrease in liver size was observed, but systemic metastases later developed and the patient died 13 years post-operatively. It was only at autopsy that the tumor was found to be a carcinoid tumor. Even from this early description, problems in future studies concerning histopathology, indolent and variable disease progression, and reporting of treatment efficacy could be anticipated.

The earliest data for cytotoxic chemotherapy of most malignancies involves the use of single agents. As new drugs became available, broad trials of various malignancies were instituted, some of which included endocrine tumors of the gastrointestinal tract. In 1963 a report appeared describing the management of disseminated carcinoid tumors by hepatic artery catheterization and 5-FU infusion.[2] Of 14 patients successfully catheterized, 11 were said to demonstrate objective improvement in liver size and most had concurrent symptomatic improvement. The authors stated in their conclusion that the "evaluation of the therapeutic usefulness [of this technique] awaits a larger, controlled study." Interestingly, although the systemic therapy of these patients has been reasonably well investigated, no such controlled studies have appeared to provide data supporting the use of intrahepatic cytotoxic chemotherapy in malignant carcinoid tumor. More recent trends toward directed chemotherapy for other hepatic neoplasms and hepatic metastases may stimulate more research in this area.

Subsequent to these studies, the activities of the alkylating agents cyclophosphamide and 1-phenylalanine (L-PAM) mustard were reported.[3,4] These studies described not only decreased tumor size in 6 of 8 courses of intravenous cyclophosphamide and 2 of 3 courses of L-PAM, but also biochemical alterations associated with successful therapy. In both series, patients experienced an exacerbation of symptoms after the drug was administered; one series reported an increase in 5-HIAA as well.

In the mid-1970s, investigators at the Mayo Clinic reported their experiences with various single agents and combination chemotherapies in the treatment of carcinoid tumor.[5] The drugs which were associated with significant numbers of responses were 5-FU (6/15 responses = 40%) and streptozotocin (3/6 responses). The antimetabolite, 5-Fluorouracil (5-FU), had been extensively tested in all other malignancies in the gastrointestinal tract, which led to its investigation in carcinoid and islet cell tumors. Streptozotocin, a nitrosourea antibiotic, was evaluated for a more specific reason: in preclinical toxicology studies, the diabetogenic potential of this drug was observed.[6] Although this toxicity predicted accurately for activities in $\beta$-cell tumors of the pancreas, the use of this drug was gradually extended to other endocrine tumors as well as to pancreatic adenocarcinoma. Although some studies failed to confirm the activity of this drug in carcinoid tumors,[7] it was rapidly incorporated into combination chemotherapy trials.

Other single agents have been evaluated in the treatment of carcinoids. A single case was reported in 1976, describing the apparent benefit after the addition of Adriamycin in a patient who had failed to respond to cyclophosphamide and methotrexate.[8] One year later, the drug DTIC (dimethyl-trianzenoimidazole-carboxamide) produced a one year response in a patient with carcinoid syndrome.[9] This drug was selected because of its activity in malignant melanoma; the presumed common neuroectodermal origin of these tumors prompted the investigators to utilize DTIC. This initial report was supported by a later study from these investigators in which 2 of 5 patients treated with DTIC demonstrated objective responses.[10]

Recently, Greek investigators reported the apparent response of a single patient with carcinoid syndrome to the synthetic antiestrogen, tamoxifen.[11] Tissue obtained by liver biopsy demonstrated "moderate" estrogen receptor activity. A multi-institutional pilot study is being conducted within the Eastern Cooperative Oncology Group to more fully elucidate the role of tamoxifen in carcinoid tumors.

Because of relatively low response rates and short durations of response with single agent chemotherapy, combination chemotherapy trials were initiated. Early reports of combinations of cyclophosphamide and methotrexate[12,13,14] were promising, but the greater activity of streptozotocin led to the preferential inclusion of this drug into combinations. The Mayo Clinic first reported responses in 6 of 9 patients treated with 5-FU and streptozotocin.[5] A similar study from the Cleveland Clinic reported objective tumor response or biochemical response in 4 of 10 patients treated with this drug combination.[15]

One of the largest trials of combination chemotherapy in the treatment of metastatic carcinoid tumor and the malignant carcinoid syndrome was conducted by investigators of the Eastern Cooperative Oncology Group (ECOG).[16] This group is comprised of investigators funded by the National Cancer Institute for the purpose of prospectively evaluating therapies of malignant neoplasms. Utilizing the information from earlier studies, a randomized comparison of 5-FU plus streptozotocin versus cyclophosphamide plus streptozotocin was performed. The objective response rates for these programs were 33% and 27% respectively. There were no apparent differences in survival relative to treatment, but marked differences in median survival were observed among sites or origin (small bowel: 29.3 months, colon: 10.1 months). These findings have implications for the analysis of subsequent trials when considering survival data and measurements of treatment efficacy.

Subsequent to these studies, the ECOG has developed a series of protocols which sequentially address issues in the therapy of patients with carcinoid tumor (Fig. 7-1). In addition to evaluating disease responses, these studies are addressing important issues in tumor biology and host responses. Preliminary data from EST 3275 were incorporated into EST 1281; neither study has been formally reported, owing to the long survival of these patients and the complex data management and statistical analysis involved in such clinical research. The importance features of these recent protocols are stringent eligibility criteria requiring:

1. that patients must be beyond hope of surgical cure
2. histologic proof of carcinoid tumor
3. measurable disease
4. significant symptoms or disability resulting from malignant disease or evidence or rapidly advancing disease
5. adequate renal, hepatic and cardiac function
6. informed consent
7. rigorous follow-up procedures for collection of response and toxicity data.

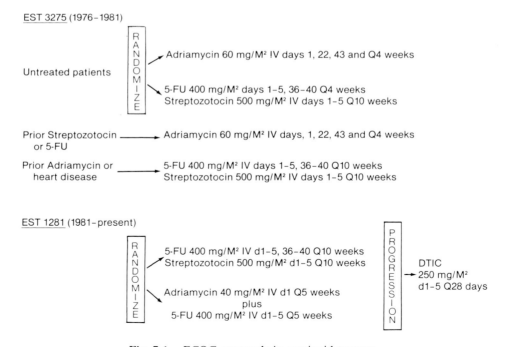

**Fig. 7-1.** ECOG protocols in carcinoid tumors.

These requirements assure that patients are only treated when they absolutely require aggressive management, in the safest and most informed manner possible.

In addition to the ECOG studies described, other groups are investigating the role of various combinations in this disease. Recently, 3 of 8 patients treated with 5-FU, Adriamycin and Cyclophosphamide in combination were documented to have objective tumor response.[17]

## SUMMARY—CARCINOID TUMORS

Only recently have rigorous prospectively controlled evaluations of cytotoxic chemotherapy become available for the treatment of patients with carcinoid tumors. In addition to the raw response data, the treating physician must be aware of the nuances involved in the treatment of these patients. The following guidelines must hold:

1. The clinician must have a good grasp of the natural history of these diseases, and should be well versed in non-chemotherapeutic management.

2. The treating physician should have intimate knowledge of the potential side effects of the various chemotherapy drugs, in particular the nephrotoxicity of streptozotocin, the myelosupression of 5-FU and the cardiotoxicity of Adriamycin.

3. The possibility of precipitating a crisis in a patient with carcinoid syndrome by cytotoxic chemotherapy should be anticipated.

Clearly, patients with aggressive symptomatic bulk disease or syndrome uncontrolled by standard non-chemotherapeutic measures should be considered for a trial of cytotoxic therapy. When possible such patients should be entered into treatment programs which will serve to advance medical knowledge. When this is not possible, physicians trained in the use of chemotherapy may choose to utilize a well-tested combination, such as 5-FU and streptozotocin in doses and schedules described in Figure 7-1.

## ISLET CELL TUMORS

Since islet cells have multiple synthetic potential, tumors arising from the endocrine pancreas may present in a variety of functioning and nonfunctioning manners. Although uncommon, the various syndromes caused by such tumors are of enormous interest to the physician. In general, as with carcinoid tumors, the initial management of these patients should include surgical debulking when feasible and non-cytotoxic therapies specific to the nature of the hormone production. Examples of this latter approach include the use of diazoxide in insulinomas and cimetidine in gastrinomas.

For the same reasons cited in the previous discussion relative to carcinoid syndrome, the data concerning the role of cytotoxic chemotherapy in these disease are difficult to interpret. Reported responses are often impossible to quantify since, until recent, criteria of response were not uniform among investigators.

The first reported chemotherapy for the treatment of a patient with a functioning islet cell tumor appeared in 1968.[18] A woman with a tumor secreting insulin, glucagon, and gastrin failed standard medical therapy and was treated with streptozotocin based on its known toxic effects to the animal $\beta$-cell. The patient sustained a prolonged, excellent remission of her disease with both decreased tumor size and hormone production. Shortly thereafter, Moertel and his co-workers at the Mayo Clinic documented 5 remissions in 8 patients with non-functioning islet cell tumors treated with streptozotocin.[19] These observations were confirmed by others in both functioning and non-functioning tumors.[20,21,22] In addition to these studies involving systemic intravenous use of streptozotocin, data has been presented demonstrating benefit for intraarterial streptozotocin in the treatment of pancreatic cholera.[23]

These observations prompted Broder and Carter in 1973 to review all patients treated with streptozotocin supplied by the National Cancer Institute.[24] This was a retrospective review; many doses and schedules were utilized. Importantly, approximately 65% of patients (25/39) with functioning tumors manifested an objective decrease in plasma hormone levels. Fifty percent (15/30) of patients with functioning tumors and with measurable bulk disease had an objective reduction in tumor mass. Additionally, 5 of 8 patients with nonfunctional tumors demonstrated objective response. Patients who responded to therapy demonstrated a median survival of 744 days compared to 298 days in non-responding patients. Although most of this improvement has been attributed to therapeutic intervention, one must always question whether patients who might have less aggressive tumors might also be more likely to respond to therapy.

Other single agents are under investigation in this disease. There are numerous reports in the literature documenting the effectiveness of DTIC in islet cell tumors.[25-30] In general, patients with glucagonomas have been most extensively evaluated; of the 15 patients reported in these studies, most had functioning glucagonomas, and all demonstrated objective remissions or stable disease for prolonged periods. The prolonged and often complete remissions in these patients have established DTIC as an initial option in patients with glucagonoma and an interesting investigational agent in other islet cell tumors.

Another nitrosourea, chlorozotocin—which has diminished nephrotoxic and emetic potential compared to streptozotocin—has been documented to produce responses in 6 of 17 patients in a Southwest Oncology Group study.[31] Given at a dose of 200 mg/M$^2$ every 6 weeks (100 mg/M$^2$ for poor-risk patients), two complete and four partial remissions were observed in both functioning (gastrin, insulin, and VIP) and non-functioning tumors. An ECOG study has also recently provided information concerning the role of Adriamycin in the therapy of islet cell tumors.[32] Twenty evaluable patients were entered; 18 had previously received 5-FU or streptozotocin. Four responses were observed with response durations of 2, 2, 6, and 30+ months.

The combination of 5-FU and streptozotocin has also been tested in islet cell tumors. Moertel documented 6/8 responses at the Mayo Clinic,[5] and individual observations confirmed the feasibility and efficacy of this regimen.[33-35] One of the largest studies reported to date was performed by the Eastern Cooperative Oncology

EST 3278 (1978–present)

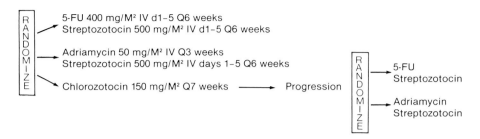

**Fig. 7-2.** ECOG protocol in islet cell carcinoma.

Group.[36] This protocol compared streptozotocin alone (500 mg/M$^2$/d × 5 days q6 weeks) to streptozotocin (500 mg/M$^2$/d × 5 days q6 weeks) plus 5-FU (400 mg/M$^2$/d × 5 days q6 weeks). Patients with functioning and non-functioning tumors were entered, although no differences were observed in response or survival between treatments. The combination showed advantage over streptozotocin alone in overall rates of response (63% vs. 36%) as well as complete response (33% vs. 12%). In general, there was concordance between responsiveness of tumor bulk and functional/hormone response. The median duration of response for all patients was 17 months; for complete responders, 24 months. A non-statistically significant survival advantage was seen for the combination (26 months) compared to streptozotocin alone (16.5 months).

The current ECOG protocol (Fig. 7-2) utilizes 5-FU plus streptozotocin as a "standard" and compares it prospectively to Adriamycin plus streptozotocin and to chlorozotocin alone. Upon progression on the latter drug, patients are randomized to either of the two combination chemotherapies. As in the protocols for carcinoid tumors, precautions are included in the protocol to include only those patients who are eligible for cytotoxic chemotherapy. In addition, stratification factors are included in statistical design—performance status, measurability, prior chemotherapy, and presence or absence of heart disease—to aid in proper selection of therapy and to facilitate data analysis. The ECOG is also seeking to confirm the activity of DTIC in patients who fail to respond to or progress on the regimens in EST 3278.

## SUMMARY—ISLET CELL TUMORS

When the treating physician has ascertained that a patient has exhausted surgical and non-chemotherapeutic options for the treatment of functional or non-functioning islet cell tumor, cytotoxic therapy should be considered. Approximately 60% of patients will evidence response to an appropriate combination chemotherapy regimen, with high numbers of complete responders and significant durations of response. The previously described 5-FU and streptozotocin regimen has been well-tested and appears to be quite active. Significant single agent activity of DTIC in glucagonomas has been documented in limited reports. Confirmation of this activity awaits larger, controlled series.

## SUMMARY

Meaningful responses with manageable toxicity have been achieved by the utilization of cytotoxic chemotherapy in endocrine-producing tumors of the gastrointestinal tract. Although the data is more convincing for functioning islet cell tumors, sufficient evidence exists to support therapy of patients with all such tumors if they are resistant to standard measures and have progressive, symptomatic disease. These patients should be entered into appropriate clinical trials when possible; if not, they should receive a recognized regimen under the direction of a qualified chemotherapist.

## REFERENCES

1. Ellis FW: Carcinoid of the rectum: Report of case of thirteen years survival: Treated with intraarterial nitrogen mustard. Cancer 10:138, 1957
2. Reed ML, Kuipers FM, Vaitkevicius VK, et al: Treatment of disseminated carcinoid tumors including hepatic artery catheterization. N Engl J Med 269:1006, 1963
3. Mengel CE, Kelly MG, Carbone PP: Clinical and biochemical effects of cyclophosphamide in patients with malignant carcinoid. Am J Med 38:396, 1965
4. Lotito CA, Mengel CE: Effect of melphalan in the malignant carcinoid syndrome. Arch Intern Med 124:36, 1969
5. Moertel CG: Clinical management of advanced gastrointestinal cancer. Cancer 36:675, 1975
6. Rakieten N, Rakieten ML, Nadkani MV: Studies of the diabetogenic action of streptozotocin (NSC-37917). Cancer Chemother Rep 29:91, 1969
7. Schein P, Kahn R, Gordon P, et al: Streptozotocin for malignant insulinomas and carcinoid tumors. Report of eight cases and review of the literature. Arch Int Med 132:555, 1973
8. Solomon A, Sonoda T, Patterson FK: Response of metastatic malignant carcinoid tumor to adriamycin. Can Treat Rep 60:273, 1976
9. Kessinger A, Foley JF, Lemon HM: Use of DTIC in the malignant carcinoid syndrome. Can Treat Rep 61:101, 1977
10. Kessinger A, Foley JF, Lemon HM: Therapy of malignant APUD cell tumors: Effectiveness of DTIC. Cancer 51:790, 1983
11. Stathopoulas GP, Karvountzis GG, Yiotis J: Tamoxifen in carcinoid syndrome. N Engl J Med 305:52, 1981
12. Mengel CE: Malignant carcinoid effect of parenteral methotrexate therapy alone and in combination with cyclophosphamide orally. Can Chemother Rep 51:239, 1967
13. Mengel CE: Therapy of the malignant carcinoid syndrome. Ann Intern Med 62:587, 1965
14. Legha SS, Valdivieso M, Nelson RS, et al: Chemotherapy of metastatic carcinoid tumors: Experiences with 32 patients and a review of the literature. Can Treat Rep 61:1699, 1977

15. Chernicoff D, Bukowski RM, Groppe CW, et al: Combination chemotherapy for islet cell carcinoma and metastatic carcinoid tumors with 5-FU and streptozotocin. Can Treat Rep 63:798, 1979
16. Moertel CG, Hanley JA: Combination chemotherapy trials for metastatic carcinoid tumor and the malignant carcinoid syndrome. Can Clin Trials 2:327, 1979
17. Jaffer A, Legha SS, Karlen DA: Combination chemotherapy of metastatic carcinoid tumors with 5FU, Adriamycin and Cytoxan (FAC) and 5FU, Adriamycin, Mitomycin and Methyl-CCNU. Proc ASCO 12/4, 1983
18. Murray-Lyon IM, Eddleston ALWF, Williams R et al: Treatment of multiple hormone producing malignant islet cell tumors with streptozotocin. Lancet 2:895, 1968
19. Moertel CG, Reitemeier RJ, Schutt AS et al: Phase II study of streptozotocin in the treatment of advanced gastrointestinal cancer. Can Chemother Rep 55:303, 1971
20. Obers K, Bostriom H, Fahrenkrus J, et al: Streptozotocin treatment of a pancreatic tumor producing VIP and gastrin associated with Verner-Morrison syndrome. Acta Med Scand 206:223, 1979
21. Lokich J, Anderson N, Rossini A, et al: Pancreatic alpha cell tumors: Case report and review of the literature. Cancer 15:45:2675, 1980
22. Stachl F, Stage G, Rehfeld JF, et al: Treatment of Zollinger Ellison syndrome with streptozotocin. N Engl J Med 294:1440, 1976
23. Kahn CR, Levy AG, Gardner JD, et al: Pancreatic cholera: Beneficial effects of treatment with streptozotocin. N Engl J Med 292:941, 1975
24. Broder LE, Carter SK: Results of therapy with streptozotocin in 52 patients. Ann Int Med 79:108, 1973
25. Kessinger A, Lemon HM, Foley JF: The glucagonoma syndrome and its management. J Surg Oncol 9:418, 1977
26. Strauss GM, Weitzman SA, Aoki TT: Dimethyltriazenoimidazole carboxamide therapy of malignant glucagonoma. Ann Int Med 90:57, 1979
27. Marynick SP, Fagadau WR, Duncan LA: Malignant glucagonoma syndrome: Response to chemotherapy. Ann Int Med 93:453, 1980
28. Prinz RA, Badrinath K, Banerji M, et al: Operative and chemotherapeutic management of malignant glucagon-producing tumors. Surgery 90:713, 1981
29. Kessinger A, Foley JF, Lemon HM: Therapy of malignant APUD cell tumors. Effectiveness of DTIC. Cancer 1:51:790, 1983
30. Awrich AE, Peetz M, Fletcher WS: Dimethyltriazenoimidazole carboxamide therapy of islet cell carcinoma of the pancreas. J Surg Oncol 17:321, 1981
31. Bukowski RM: Chemotherapy of islet cell carcinoma with chlorozotocin. A SWOG study. Proc ASCO 90, 1982
32. Moertel CG, Lavin PT, Hahn RG: Phase II trial of doxorubicin therapy for advanced islet cell carcinoma. Can Treat Rep 66:1567, 1982
33. Chernicoff D, Bukowski RM, Groppe CW Jr, Hewlett JS: Combination chemotherapy for islet cell carcinoma and metastatic carcinoid tumors with 5-fluorouracil and streptozotocin. Can Treat Rep 63:795, 1979
34. Khandekar JD, Over D, Miller HJ, Vick NA: Neurologic involvement in glucagonoma syndrome: Response to combination chemotherapy with 5-fluorouracil and streptozotocin. Cancer 44:2014, 1979
35. Awrich A, Fletcher WS, Klotz JH, et al: 5-FU versus combination therapy with tubercidin, streptozotocin, and 5-FU in the treatment of pancreatic carcinomas: COG protocol 7230. J Surg Oncol 12:267, 1979
36. Moertel CG, Hanley JA, Johnson LA: Streptozotocin alone compared with streptozotocin plus fluorouracil in the treatment of advanced islet cell carcinoma. N Engl J Med 303:1189, 1980

# 8 | Surgical Approaches to Endocrine-Producing Tumors of the Gastrointestinal Tract

*David McFadden*
*Bernard M. Jaffe*

## INTRODUCTION

Despite the differences among endocrine-producing tumors of the gastrointestinal tract, the objectives in their surgical management are identical, namely, to:

1. establish the diagnosis histologically
2. cure the symptoms
3. prevent induced complications
4. manage the neoplasms themselves

As discussed in the individual chapters, the symptoms and complications are specific for each of the tumors; consequently, no overriding generalizations are appropriate. In contrast, the surgical approaches to management of the tumors themselves share several important features; these include:

1. obviously, the primary goal is total tumor excision
2. it is difficult to distinguish benignancy from malignancy on histologic criteria alone

139

3. in the presence of metastases, debulking may be appropriate
4. there is no definite relationship between tumor mass and the intensity of symptoms
5. no histologic characteristics are predictive of survival
6. if control of the tumor is not possible, surgery may be directed against the responsive end-organ

This chapter will review the specific surgical approaches to each of the endocrine-producing tumors of the gastrointestinal tract, focusing on the direct applications to each of the lesions themselves.

## GASTRINOMAS

In 1955 Zollinger and Ellison[1] reported two patients whose clinical syndrome consisted of intractable peptic ulceration severe enough to warrant total gastrectomy, severe hypersecretion of gastric hydrochloric acid, and pancreatic islet cell tumors morphologically different from insulin-secreting B-cell lesions. Although Zollinger and Ellison originally postulated an "ulcerogenic humoral factor" it was Gregory and associates[2] who first suggested and later proved[3] that these tumors produce gastrin. The development of a radioimmunoassay for gastrin[4] facilitated both the diagnosis and therapeutic monitoring of these patients. Elevated circulating gastrin leads to a continuous parietal cell stimulation with resultant gastric hyperacidity as well as trophic stimulation of the parietal cell mass.[5] The incidence of the syndrome is estimated as between 0.1 and 1% of patients with peptic ulcer disease,[6] and approximately 200–400 new cases are reported annually in the United States and Canada.[7] Males have a slight predominance over females, and although all ages are affected, the majority of patients are young, in the 3rd through 5th decades.[6,8] Since the presentation is often identical to that of routine peptic ulcer disease, there has generally been a 3–5 year delay in establishing the diagnosis.[9]

Surgical management of gastrinoma includes treatment of the associated ulcer complications. Abdominal pain is the most common symptom, present in 75% of patients, and diarrhea, often debilitating, is seen in 8–40% of patients.[8,9] The emergent complications of peptic ulcer disease are more common in Zollinger–Ellison Syndrome (ZES), particularly upper gastrointestinal hemorrhage and hematemesis. Ulcers are usually solitary, small, and located in the first portion of the duodenum. About one-fourth of ulcers are multiple or located distal to the proximal duodenum, with 11% in the jejunum.[10] Up to 25% of ZES patients will not present with ulceration at time of diagnosis. The findings of gastric rugal hypertrophy, rapid gastric emptying, multiple or distally located ulcers, or ulcers in patients less than 25 years of age[11] are all clues to the presence of gastrinoma. Recurrent peptic ulcer after surgical therapy and peptic ulcer disease refractory to medical management should also alert the clinician. Although the techniques for the diagnosis of gastrinomas are detailed in Chapter 2, the measurement of serum gastrin is critical. Hypergastrinemic, hypersecretory states other than ZES include retained gastric antrum, gastric outlet obstruction, renal failure, antral G-cell hyperplasia, and the short-bowel syndrome.[5,6,9] Multiple Endocrine Neoplasia Syndrome Type I (MEN I, or Wermer's Syndrome) has associated gastrinoma or gastrin-secreting islet cell hyperplasia in 40–60% of cases,[6] and overall 25% of ZES patients have MEN I. The possibility of gastrinoma should be suspected in all first-degree members of families with MEN I, especially those with previous parathyroid disorders.

Sixty percent of gastrinomas are malignant with over one-half of them metastatic at time of surgery.[8,11] Recent reviewers, using aggressive diagnostic intervention, have reported somewhat lower incidences of metastases.[12-14] Metastases from malignant gastrinomas commonly involve lymph nodes in the paraduodenal, parapancreatic, inferior gastric, and subplyoric areas. The liver, spleen, bone, mediastinum, peritoneum, and skin are also recognized sites of metastasis. Tumors may be multiple or solitory benign adenomas (30%) or islet cell hyperplasia in 1–10%[6-8] of cases. Islet cell hyperplasia, although sometimes the only pathologic finding, may be a result rather than a cause of ZES, as gastrinomas are recognized later in many of the patients. Duodenal tumors are found in 13% of patients,[8,15] with nearly one-half solitary and nonmetastatic. Associated pancreatic tumors are found in 23% of patients with duodenal tumors.[15]

Attempts at preoperative localization are important aspects of surgical care. Unfortunately, the majority of radiographic techniques fail to locate many gastrinomas. Ultrasonic scanning is able to detect primary pancreatic gastrinomas in only 28% of patients,[9,16] but its safety and ease warrants its initial usage. CT scanning has been reported diagnostic in up to 81% of patients[17] but two large reviews revealed only 18–22% detection rates.[18,19] Despite being vascular tumors, gastrinomas are angiographically demonstrated in less than 20% of attempts,[9,20] although this technique is reported as better than ultrasound or CT scanning in detecting hepatic metastases.[21] Hepatic isotopic scanning, although not prospectively evaluated, is recommended to supplement the search for metastases. Pancreatic venous sampling (PVS) for serial gastrin assays has been successful in up to 94% of cases.[20,22] This technique is preferred if no metastatic disease is found and a curative resection is anticipated.

The management of patients with the ZES is controversial and is clearly still evolving. Prior to the advent of histamine receptor antagonist therapy, the accepted treatment of choice was removal of the target organ by total gastrectomy. The combination of a high frequency of metastatic disease, multiplicity of tumors, inability to preoperatively localize tumors, and undetectable tumors in up to 48% of explorations[9,23] has led most surgeons to perform total gastrectomy. With the development of better methods to control gastric secretion, many have advocated a "chemical gastrectomy" as the preferred therapy, citing high surgical mortality and significant morbidity.[24] Although $H_2$-receptor antagonists have no effect on the malignancy, the decision to place patients on lifetime medication is defended by many physicians[9,24,25] despite an overall expected 33% failure rate[26]; failure often necessitates emergency surgical treatment.[27] The frequent necessity to serially increase the dosage of cimetidine with a concomitant increase in side effects (gynecomastia, impotency) may be obviated by the newer histamine receptor antagonists, which are reported to be more effective and safer than cimetidine.[11,28] $H_2$-receptor antagonist therapy is certainly an effective means for perioperative control and stabilization of the gastrinoma patient, but it cannot be recommended as the long-term treatment of choice for this disease because of the high failure rate, the incidence of side effects and the requirement for a lifetime dependency even in compliant, well-motivated patients.

The surgical debate concerning ZES revolves around extirpative tumor surgery versus total gastrectomy. Lesser gastric resections and vagotomy[29] have not been prospectively evaluated but preliminary and retrospective data suggest a lower overall efficiency. Proponents of extirpative tumor surgery[17,25,30-35] cite the possibility of cure for these patients without a lifetime of medication or potential nutritional difficulty. Unfortunately, surgical cures are possible in less than 20% of patients explored[13] and in one-half of "curatively resected" patients, the disease recurs.[24] Surgical mortality rates and projected survival figures for patients whose tumors are resected and those treated by total gastrectomy do not differ significantly; in the former group, recurrence mandates further surgery or the onus of lifetime medical therapy.

Our current approach to management consists of preoperative control of gastric acid secretion with an $H_2$-receptor antagonist followed by vigorous localization attempts. All patients of suitable surgical risk are explored and obvious metastases are searched for and confirmed by biopsy. The pancreas and duodenum are mobilized by a Kocher manuever and the peritoneum inferior to the pancreas is incised to allow full palpation of the gland. If an apparent, solitary, nonmetastatic tumor of the distal pancreas is found, we recommend a distal pancreatectomy and close follow-up of the patient using serial gastrin determinations; this circumstance is quite rare. If hypergastrinemia persists or recurs we perform a total gastrectomy. The remaining (and overwhelming majority of patients) receive a total gastrectomy with Roux-en-Y esophagojejunostomy. Recent mortality figures for this procedure in the hands of experienced surgeons average less than 3%, with minimal nutritional morbidity.[7,8,13,33] Although tumor regression[36] and increased survival in patients with metastatic disease[15] have been reported after total gastrectomy, we do not feel these are relevant arguments. Postoperative chemotherapy is considered for patients with obvious metastatic disease.

Survival projections vary widely and are subject to the unpredictable, often indolent, nature of the growth of these tumors as well as the therapy applied. In general, patients with MEN I fare considerably worse than do patients with isolated gastrinomas. Overall, 10-year survival rates approaching 60% are reported after total gastrectomy.[17] Death as a result of malignancy occurs in only 27–50% of patients with gastrinomas.[15,37]

# INSULINOMAS

Insulin-secreting tumors of the pancreas have been recognized since 1927, when Roscoe Graham first described the successful removal of an insulinoma.[38] Eleven years later Whipple[39] described the classic triad of findings associated with the syndrome: symptoms of insulin shock with fasting, fasting blood sugars less than one-half of normal, and relief of symptoms upon infusion of glucose. The capability at measuring plasma insulin levels by radioimmunoassay, developed by Yalow and Berson in 1959,[40] confirms the hyperinsulinemic state of the patients and simplifies the clinical diagnosis. Insulinomas are the second most frequently described functioning pancreatic islet cell tumor and approximately 1500 cases had been described by 1980. Sixty percent of the patients are women and the average age at the time of diagnosis is 45 years of age[41] but newborns[42] and octogenarians are known to be affected.

The clinical findings associated with insulinomas are predominantly neuropsychiatric and are related to the hypoglycemic effects on the nervous system. Because of this, up to 20% of patients[43] are initially treated for these disturbances leading to delays in accurate diagnosis averaging 32.5 months.[44] Over 90% of patients[8] episodically suffer from such neuropyschiatric symptoms as syncope, confusion, coma, dizziness, visual changes, personality changes, and epilepsy. Autonomic symptoms are secondary to hypoglycemia-induced stimulation of the sympathetic nervous system leading to weakness, sweating, tremors, palpitations, and hunger. To obviate symptoms, some patients eat frequently and obesity is present in 15–48%.[41,43]

The extent of attempts at preoperative localization is controversial, since 76 to 97%[41,45] of tumors are palpable at surgery. Methods available include ultrasound and computerized tomography, which are valuable for large pancreatic tumors; however, more than 60% of solitary insulinomas are less than 1.5 cm in size.[46] Selective arteriographic techniques have been reported successful in 29%[47] to 90%[48] of cases with a 5% false-positive rate. Percutaneous selective pancreatic vein catheterization (PCV) with serial plasma collection for insulin assay has been used with over 92% success.[47-49]

Eighty per cent of insulinomas are solitary and benign, with a uniform distribution throughout the pancreas.[41,6,50] Approximately 10% of patients have multiple adenomas and up to 50% of these patients have Multiple Endocrine Neoplasia Type I (MEN).[44] Between 10 and 15% of patients have malignant insulinomas of which one-third have metastasized to the liver or lymph nodes at time of diagnosis.[41] Islet cell hyperplasia is reported in up to 6.5%[41,43] of adult patients, whereas diffuse pancreatic islet disease is seen in over three-fourths of infants and over one-fourth of children with pancreatic hypoglycemia.[42] Ectopic insulinomas, seen in up to 2.6% of patients,[45] are usually found in peripancreatic tissue, the splenic hilum, or the duodenal submucosa.

The preoperative administration of diazoxide is controversial, as are all other aspects of insulinoma management. In adults, diazoxide may afford good control of symptoms in 50 to 100% of patients,[41,51] with side effects necessitating discontinuation in 10%. The advantage to the surgeon in using preoperative diazoxide is that it demonstrates before surgery if this drug will be therapeutic in case the exploration is negative. This allows the surgeon time for further investigation (by PCV or repeated angiography) of a symptomatically controlled patient before reoperation. Disadvantages of its use include its frequency of side effects and its untoward influence on glucose levels as an intraoperative resectional aide.

The optimal surgical approach to these tumors necessitates thorough preoperative preparation and frequent intraoperative measurements of serum glucose to maintain levels of at least 60 mg/dl.[52] Many factors affect serum glucose during surgery, including the anesthetic agent employed, manipulation of the tumor, and the amount of intravenously administered glucose. The controversy concerning the usefulness of serial levels of serum glucose as an indicator of tumor resection is discussed below, but no patient should be allowed to suffer further hypoglycemic damage intraoperatively.

Wide operative exposure is the key to successful pancreatic exploration. A bilateral subcostal or generous midline incision suffices in most patients. The liver and periportal lymph nodes should be examined carefully for metastases and biopsied if suspicious. If a tumor has been localized preoperatively, it is still necessary to perform a complete pancreatic exploration, since the incidence of multiple tumors is 10%.[53] A Kocher manuever is performed to examine the pancreatic head by incising the peritoneum lateral to the duodenum, and mobilizing the pancreas and duodenum to the aorta. The body and tail of the pancreas are exposed by dividing the gastrocolic omentum and elevating the stomach to reveal the anterior pancreatic surface. The peritoneum at the inferior margin of the pancreas should be incised to allow mobilization of the body and tail. A careful bimanual palpation of the gland is then performed. Most lesions are palpably more firm than the surrounding pancreatic tissue and when close to the surface, may appear reddishbrown.

The preferred treatment for solitary insulinomas is simple enucleation. A dissection plane should be gently created immediately adjacent to the tumor to avoid ductal or vascular damage. Up to 75% of tumors can be managed safely this way.[45] For multiple lesions of the body and tail, a distal pancreatectomy should be performed although some authors recommend distal resection even for single tumors of the body or tail to prevent recurrence due to unsuspected multiple adenomas. A T-tube may be placed in the common bile duct to aid in enucleation of pancreatic head tumors.

Malignant insulinomas are to be treated as any pancreatic carcinoma. Distal pancreatectomy should be performed for body and tail tumors. Total pancreatectomy or radical pancreaticoduodenectomy is reserved for malignant tumors of the head or uncinate process. If a curative resection is not possible, as much as possible of the primary tumor and the metastases should be resected for palliation,[52,54] although some clinicians recommend only biliary and gastroenteric bypass with postoperative streptozotocin.

Using the above techniques, up to 25% of insulinomas will not be detected. Under those circumstances, we recommend mobilization of the spleen to examine the pancreatic tail and splenic hilum for tumor. A small duodenotomy should be performed to detect any submucosal or periduodenal tumors. Other areas to be investigated include the stomach and retroperitoneum.[46] Careful attention to the head of the gland is important, as one large review[55] reported 54% of occult tumors in the pancreatic head; nonetheless, "blind" pancreaticoduodenectomies are to be condemned. Numerous intraoperative methods of locating an occult insulinoma have been suggested, including ultrasound,[56,57] intraarterial toluidine blue,[58] and cholangiopancreatography.[41] Rapid radioimmunoassay of serial pancreatic venous blood for insulin levels has been successfully performed,[59] but this technique is generally unavailable. If after these maneuvers, no tumor is found, serial resections of the tail and body of the pancreas is recommended with repeated pathological examination and blood glucose monitoring. As much as 90% of the pancreas can be resected in this fashion if necessary, and 46 to 90% of patients benefit,[41,60] including those with diffuse islet cell hyperplasia. The expected rise in blood glucose after tumor resection is not seen in up to 23% of cases,[61] severely limiting the utility of this technique. However, it remains the quickest, most easily performed, and most clinically available means to confirm resection of occult insulinoma intraoperatively. A glucose-controlled insulin and glucose infusion system (Biostator System, Miles Laboratories Inc., Elkhart, Ind.) has been used to successfully monitor and localize tumors in these patients[62,63] but its expense and the requirement for a trained technician limit its use at present.

In infants and children, diffuse islet cell hyperplasia and nesidioblastosis are seen much more frequently than local adenomas. Prompt subtotal or total pancreatectomies are nearly always necessary in these patients[42,64] to avoid permanent neurological damage or mental retardation.

Complications of surgery for insulinoma have been reported in up to 55% of patients[45] and are related to the type of surgery as well as its metabolic effects. Major complications include fistulae, pseudocysts, pancreatitis, and sepsis. Diabetes is seen postoperatively in 10% of patients, although temporary hyperglycemia is very common. Peptic ulcer disease later develops in one-third of patients.[46] Reoperation for persistent or recurrent hypoglycemia is required in about 15% of patients but tumors are found in only 35% of reexplored patients.[55] Mortality rates have declined in recent reports from the 11% average reported by Stefanini[41] presumably due to better preoperative management. Death is usually secondary to pancreatitis or sepsis.

If hypoglycemia recurs or persists after subtotal pancreatic resection, control with diazoxide is recommended while intensive attempts at localization by PCV or repeated arteriography are instituted. Growth rate data fail to indicate any advantage to waiting for prolonged periods before reoperation, unless repeated localization attempts fail and the patient is comfortably controlled on diazoxide.[55] Malignant tumors that cannot be resected for cure are best treated with streptozotocin[35] and diazoxide, if necessary. Five-year survival rates of 33% are reported.[43]

## GLUCAGONOMAS

Although clinically suspected by Becker and associates[65] over 40 years ago, it was not until McGavran et al. in 1966[66] and Mallison and colleagues in 1974[67] distinguished glucagon-secreting islet cell tumors of the pancreas as a recognizable clinical entity. It is sometime referred to as the hyperglycemic, cutaneous syndrome[68] because of its dominant clinical features. The skin rash, known as necrolytic migratory erythema, is specific to the disease and is usually accompanied by weight loss, normochromic normocytic anemia, cheilosis, and diabetes mellitus.[69,70] Plasma glucagon levels, as measured by radioimmunoassay, are generally elevated above 500 pg/ml,[71] and serial measurements afford an excellent means of follow-up. Only about 60 cases have been reported in the literature, with the majority of patients being women in the 5th to 7th decades of life. A familial hyperglucagenemic syndrome has been reported[72] with autosomally dominant transmission. Once suspected, preoperative localization via arteriography, CT scanning, and ultrasonography may be technically helpful, and exact localization has been accomplished by selective pancreatic vein catheterization and blood sampling for glucagon analysis.[73]

Because of the indolent nature of the symptoms and poor physician recognition, late diagnosis has been the rule. Three quarters of the patients explored already have metastatic disease.[69] The majority of tumors in one large review[74] were large (more than 3 cm in diameter) and found in the body or tail of the gland; less than one-third were suitable for an attempt at curative resection. Of these tumors resected for cure, 20% later recurred. Metastases are most commonly found in the liver, lymph nodes, adrenal glands, and the spine. Early laparotomy with an attempt at curative pancreatic resection is the recommended treatment for these patients[69,74] and in the presence of metastatic disease, surgical debulking of the primary tumor and metastases is strongly suggested for symptomatic control. The time course of the disease is protracted, despite the presence of metastases,[75] and asymptomatic long-term survivors have been reported.[76] Islet cell hyperplasia, usually in multiple and small sites, rarely produce this syndrome[34,77] and a good response to subtotal distal pancreatectomy has been reported.[78]

Chemotherapy for the malignant glucagonoma syndrome is suggested for poor-risk surgical patients, for those with unresectable disease, and for recurrence. Streptozotocin has had limited success[35] but recent reports of the success of dimethyltriazenoimidaxole carboxamide (DTIC) against this tumor look hopeful.[69,79]

## SOMATOSTATINOMAS

Somatostatin, a tetradecapeptide discovered in 1973[80] and localized to pancreatic islet D cells in 1975,[81] has well-characterized suppressive effects on TSH, GH, insulin, glucagon, gastrin, pepsin, secretin, and exocrine pancreatic secretion, as well as depressive effects on intestinal and gallbladder motility.[50] Less than 4 years after discovery of the hormone, malignant islet cell tumors with high somatostatin content were incidentally discovered at cholecystectomy in both the United States[82] and Europe.[83] At present, there are only 14 reported cases in the literature, all histologically malignant, and 10 of these cases had metastasized by the time of initial laparotomy.[84,85] Two-thirds of the pancreatic tumors were localized within the pancreatic head, and all but one were single tumors. The classic triad of symptoms as described by Krejs et al.[86] of gallstones, diabetes mellitus, and diarrhea with steatorrhea are seen in over one-half of patients; however, these manitations are so nonspecific and vague that long delays in diagnosis are usual, up to 15 years in one case.[87] It is of note that both reported cases of duodenal tumors were asymptomatic.[88,89] Five of the tumors were localized preoperatively by angiography,[85] but experience with this technique is limited.

Treatment has ranged from simple enucleation to radical pancreaticoduodenectomy. The use of postoperative streptozotocin has been favorably reported.[34] Because of the evidence that all of these tumors are malignant, total extirpative surgery is recommended, if possible. Palliative resection of symptomatic metastases is also suggested due to the resolution of symptoms in resected patients, and the indolent, albeit progressive, growth of these tumors. Postoperative serum somatostatin levels afford an effective means of defecting recurrence.

## DIARRHEAGENIC TUMORS

Since the initial report by Verner and Morrison[90] of an islet cell tumor producing symptoms of refractory diarrhea, approximately 100 cases have been reported in the literature[91,92] and referred to as the Verner–Morrison Syndrome, VIPoma, pancreatic cholera, and the watery diarrhea, hypokalemia, achlorhydria (WDHA) syndrome. It seems likely that this is a heterogeneous set of tumors and various circulating agents have been etiologically implicated, including prostaglandins[93] and pancreatic polypeptide.[94,95] However, it appears that the majority of these patients have elevated plasma levels of vasoactive intestinal polypeptide (VIP)[92,96] and plasma levels, as measured by RIA,[97] greater than 50 pmol per liter generally indicate the presence of a tumor.[98]

The clinical features of profuse watery diarrhea, hypokalemia, hypochlorhydria, flushing, hyperglycemia, and hypercalcemia are so characteristic that the diagnosis is generally made on clinical grounds alone. Once the diagnosis is made, surgical removal is the treatment of choice, since even histologically benign adenomas have caused mortalities from their metabolic effects.[92] In fact, the commonest cause of death in this syndrome is chronic renal failure due to dehydration and hypokalemic vascular nephropathy. Thus, every attempt must be made to excise all the tumor. Preoperative correction of metabolic derangements and volume deficits is strongly recommended, and some clinicians advocate the use of preoperative steroids[99,100] and/or indomethacin[101] to facilitate preparation. Perioperative use of antacids or $H_2$-blockers is recommended because of reported cases of rebound hyperchlorhydria and gastrointestinal bleeding after surgery.[92] Preoperative localization of these generally solitary tumors is suggested since 10 to 15% of these tumors are extrapancreatic in origin; the adrenals, sympathetic chain, and retroperitoreum are additional sites, especially in children, where 70% of these tumors are ganglioneuroblastomas. Ultrasound,[16] CT scanning,[100] and arteriography[92] have all been used with success. One large review cited angiography as most effective.[92] Between 37[91] and 61%[102] of these tumors are malignant with 40% manifesting hepatic and/or nodal metastases at initial laparotomy. In contrast, only 10% of extra-pancreatic tumors were found to be metastatic at laparotomy.[92]

The pancreatic body and tail have been the site of 80% of palpable tumors[103] with distal pancreatectomies the most widely performed procedure in this circumstance. Radical pancreaticoduodenectomies must be reserved for resectable tumors of the head or uncinate process. Nonpalpable islet cell hyperplasia has been reported in up to 20% of patients[91] and although clinical experience is limited, distal or 75% pancreatectomy to the margin of the superior mesenteric vessels has been successfully utilized[99,100]; up to 73% of these patients respond.[91] Despite the indolent growth characteristics of these tumors, their devastating metabolic consequences warrant surgical debulking of the tumor and metastases when feasible. Outstanding long-term results of debulking have been reported.[103] Postoperative streptozotocin, either alone or combined with 5-FU, has been successfully utilized in these patients and is recommended for high-risk surgical patients or those with known metastatic disease.[35,104] Postoperative VIP levels should be used for monitoring recurrence.

## CARCINOID TUMORS

Over 75 years ago Oberndorfer[105] first used the term "Karzinoide" to describe an unusual ileal tumor. The malignant propensity of these tumors was later recognized and Thorson, in 1954,[106] first delineated the functional aspects of carcinoids and described the malignant carcinoid syndrome. Williams and Sandler[107] divided these tumors according to embryologic origin as foregut, midgut, and hindgut tumors. Foregut carcinoids are argentaffin negative and argyrophil positive and elaborate 5-hydroxytryptophan, a serotonin precursor, as their primary product.[108] Foregut tumors, such as bronchial and gastric carcinoids, produce a variant of the classic carcinoid syndrome with intense flushing, lacrimation, diaphoresis, vomiting, and bronchospasm as salient features. Midgut carcinoids are both argyrophil and argentaffin positive and secrete serotonin, 5-hydroxytryptamine, as a prime mediator of the classic carcinoid syndrome which consists of flushing, hypotension, bronchoconstriction, and right-sided cardiac lesions.[108,109] Other substances that have been associated with the carcinoid syndrome include histamine, catecholamines, kinins, prostaglandins, substance P, and motilin.[110] Hindgut tumors are both argyrophil and argentaffin negative and generally produce no specific metabolically active substance.

Over 4000 reports of carcinoid tumors have been recorded[111] with over 90% originating in the gastrointestinal tract; carcinoids represent 1.5% of gastrointestinal neoplasms.[110] Although reported in every enteric organ, the major sites of involvement are the appendix, small bowel, and rectum. Bronchial and ovarian carcinoids are also reported in significant numbers. The carcinoid syndrome is seen in up to 30% of patients with small intestinal tumors[112] but the incidence of syndrome from all carcinoid tumors is between 3 and 4%. The presence of the syndrome usually indicates functioning hepatic metastases, but its presence is seen in less than one-half of patients with metastatic tumors.[110,111] Recently, patients without liver metastases have been shown to have the carcinoid syndrome,[113] perhaps due to retroperitoneal tumor implants with systemic venous drainage. The development of a radioimmunoassay for serotonin[114] has facilitated the diagnosis as well as serial therapeutic monitoring of these patients. In the absence of the carcinoid syndrome, symptoms relative to mass effect and site of origin predominate, although most series also include a substantial proportion of autopsy and incidental cases.

Multiplicity of carcinoids has been reported in 21 to 23% of small bowel tumors[101,115,116]; lower but still significant incidences are noted with carcinoids originating from other sites. Associated noncarcinoid malignancies are seen in up to 45% of patients,[117] with about one-half of these cancers being intraabdominal; the most common lesion is adenocarcinoma of the colon. These significant associations necessitate a thorough examination of the abdomen in all patients explored for carcinoid tumors. Another frequent association is that of peptic ulcer disease, seen in up to one-fourth of patients.[108,118]

The overall poor response of these tumors to chemotherapy and radiotherapy makes surgical extirpation the treatment of choice for all carcinoid tumors. Thus, anesthesia may be a significant problem. Anesthetic management of patients with functioning carcinoid tumors may require the use of preoperative promethazine to inhibit release of vasoactive substances.[110] The use of aprotinin, epsilon-aminocaproic acid (Amicar), and somatostatin have all been reported to reduce the instances of bradykininogenic signs caused by induction of anesthesia. Appropriate blocking agents and hydration to expand the extracellular fluid volume add to the safety of intraoperative management.

## Gastroduodenal Carcinoids

Comprising only 2% of all gastrointestinal carcinoids,[119] these foregut tumors are usually found in the distal stomach or proximal duodenum.[120] The carcinoid syndrome is seen in up to 28% of these patients and up to three-fourths of patients have documented upper gastrointestinal bleeding.[121] Other symptoms include epigastric pain, vomiting, and weight loss. Barium studies and endoscopic evoluation often locate the tumor,[109] commonly ulcerated or with an associated peptic ulcer.[111] For tumors less than 1 cm in size, lymphatic metastases have been demonstrated in only 2.4% of tumors[122] and local excision can be performed safely. For larger gastric tumors, subtotal gastrectomy with omentectomy is necessary.[109] Larger duodenal tumors require pancreaticoduodenectomy. As with all carcinoid tumors, metastatic deposits should be resected if possible due to their slow growth and to provide symptomatic palliation. Overall, 5-year survival rates for this site are 52%.[119]

## Pancreatic Carcinoids

The pancreas is an extremely uncommon site for primary carcinoid involvement and no such case was included in one review of over 2500 cases.[119] Affected patients are generally diagnosed late but manifest the carcinoid syndrome or abdominal pain associated with a palpable mass. Standard resectional techniques for malignant tumors of the pancreas should be performed, along with resection of accessible metastases. The prophylactic creation of a biliary–enteric bypass and a gastroenterostomy for large tumors is also suggested for long-term palliation.

## Small Intestinal Carcinoids

The small intestine is the second most common site of gastrointestinal carcinoid tumors[119] with over 1000 cases reported[112]; the majority of these arise in the distal ileum. Common symptoms include abdominal pain, diarrhea, weight loss, and rectal bleeding.[122] Small bowel carcinoids also tend to produce a dense fibroplastic reaction with contraction and fibrosis leading to bowel obstruction in up to 50% of patients. A unique mesenteric angiopathy with intestinal gangrene has also been reported.[123] Small bowel carcinoids are the most frequently associated with multiple tumors and other malignancies, incidences for which average 30%.[112,117,124] Only 40% are localized at time of diagnosis, while a similar percentage of patients present with the carcinoid syndrome.

Even small tumors less than 1 cm have been shown to have lymphatic invasion in 19% of cases.[112,122] This necessitates generous small bowel excision with resection of adjacent mesentery.[112,117,121,125,126] A careful search for multiple tumors and associated malignancies must also be performed. Every effort should be made to resect all visible tumor, including mesenteric, omental, and localized liver metastases.[109,117,127] Distal ileal lesions require ileo-right colectomy to adequately remove the lymphatic drainage, and it should be noted that local recurrence with bowel obstruction is the leading cause of late morbidity in these patients.[117] Hepatic resection of localized metastases has led to symptomatic responses lasting an average of 3 years,[128] considerably longer than either hepatic artery ligation, embolization, or infusion of chemotherapeutic agents.[128-130] The latter therapeutic alternatives are recommended in poor risk patients and those with unresectable metastases. Overall 5-year survival rate average 54%[119] and fall to 21% in the presence of liver metastases.[125]

## Appendiceal Carcinoids

The appendix is the most common site of origin of carcinoid tumors. These lesions comprise 30 to 40% of all reported cases.[119,122] Carcinoids are also the most common tumor of the appendix, seen in approximately 0.3% of appendices[121]; the majority of these tumors are discovered incidentally at laparotomy or autopsy. As described by Beaton et al.,[111] other clinical settings of appendiceal carcinoids include acute appendicitis (in which the tumor is causative in less than one-third of the association), chronic right lower quadrant pain, and the malignant carcinoid syndrome, only six cases of which had been reported by 1981. It was Moertel and colleagues' large review of these tumors[131] that led to the modern, albeit controversial, approach to their surgical management. Briefly stated, tumors less than 2 cm in size and without gross invasive characteristics (involvement of cecum, etc.) can be treated by simple appendectomy. Larger and invasive tumors necessitate a formal right hemicolectomy. Other observers have reported metastatic disease in tumors between 1 and 2 cm in diameter and recommend 1 cm as the upper size limit for removal by simple appendectomy. Despite these data, most clinicians use the 2-cm rule for lesions without gross invasion or extension.[121,126,132] Associated malignancies occur in up to 28% of cases.[133] The overall five year survival rates approach 99%.[119]

## Colonic Carcinoids

Carcinoid tumors of the colon, exclusive of the appendix and rectum, account for 7% of all carcinoid tumors, with an overall 5-year survival rate of 52%.[119] Approximately one-third arise in the cecum and three-fourths in the right colon,[134] presumably due to the higher concentration of EC cells present. Considered by most reviewers to have the highest malignant potential of all carcinoids,[111,135] these tumors generally present with signs and symptoms identical to colonic adenocarcinoma and average 4.9 cm in size at the time of diagnosis.[134] Only 4% are multiple but 60% have metastasized when diagnosed.[119,134] Treatment consists of standard cancer resection for the affected area of the colon with debulking of unresectable, metastatic deposits if present. Liver resection for hepatic metastases has also been suggested; significant improvement in symptoms and survival have been reported.[127,128]

## Rectal Carcinoids

The rectum is the third most common site of gastrointestinal carcinoids, comprising 12 to 15% of these tumors.[119] Carcinoids are second in frequency to adenomatous polyps among tumors of the rectum.[124] Approximately 60% are palpable on rectal exam and over 90% can be visualizable at sigmidoscopy.[121] Symptoms of rectal pain, bleeding, and tenesmus are common, but the carcinoid syndrome is very rare, even in the presence of widely metastatic disease. A careful examination of the patient is required, as up to 10% of patients have synchronous anorectal carcinomas and up to one-third have other associated malignancy.[121] Overall, 85% of tumors are localized at time of diagnosis and 5-year survival rates of 83% have been reported.[119] Peskin and Orloff[136] noted a 4% incidence of invasion or metastasis in tumors less than 2 cm versus 80% for larger carcinoids. Consequently, they recommended simple excision for the tumors less than 2 cm, and either abdominoperineal or low anterior resection for the larger lesions. They have reported a 76% 5-year survival rate using these criteria.[137] Most current clinicians recommend simple excision of tumors less than 2 cm in size followed by formal abdominoperineal or low anterior resection if pathological examination reveals muscular invasion.[109,111,124,125] Larger tumors require cancer resection procedures without prior excision.

## REFERENCES

1. Zollinger RM, Ellison EH: Primary peptic ulcerations of the jejunum associated with islet cell tumors of the pancreas. Ann Surg 142:709, 1955
2. Gregory RA, French JM, Sircus W, Tracy HJ: Extraction of a gastrin-like substance from a pancreatic tumor in a case of ZES. Lancet 1:1045, 1960
3. Gregory RA, Tracy HJ. A note on the gastrin-like stimulant present in ZE tumors. Gut 5:115, 1964
4. McGuigan JE, Trudeau WL: Immunochemical measurement of elevated levels of gas-

trin in the serum of patients with pancreatic tumors of the ZE variety. N Eng J Med 278:1308, 1968

5. Stadil F: Gastrinomas. p. 729. In: Gastrointestinal Hormones. Glass GB, Ed. New York: Raven Press, 1980

6. McGuigan JE: The Zollinger–Ellison Syndrome. P. 693. In: Gastrointestinal Disease. Sleisenger M, Fortran J, Eds. Philadelphia: WB Saunders, 1983

7. Thompson JC: Zollinger–Ellison Syndrome. P. 263. In: Gastrointestinal Surgery, Najarian JC and Delancey JP, Eds. Miami: Symposia Specialists, 1979

8. Dooner J, Harrison RC, Cleator IGM: Gastrin secreting tumors. Contemp Surg 18:35, 1981

9. Jensen RT, Gardner JD, Raufman JP, Pandol SJ, Doppman JL, Collen MJ: Zollinger–Ellison Syndrome: Current Concepts and Management. NIH Conference. Ann Int Med 98:59, 1983

10. Ellison EH, Wilson SD: The ZES: Reappraissal and evaluation of 260 registered cases. Ann Surg 160:512, 1964

11. Modlin IM, Brennan MF: The diagnosis and management of gastrinoma. Surg Gynec Obst 158:97, 1984

12. Zollinger RM, Ellison EC, Fabri PJ, Johnson J, Sparks J, Carey L: Primary peptic ulcerations of the jejunum associated with islet cell tumors; Twenty-five-year appraisal. Ann Surg 192:422, 1980

13. Deveney CW, Deveney KS, Way LW: The Zollinger–Ellison Syndrome—23 years later. Ann Surg 188:384, 1978

14. Thompson JC, Lewis BG, Weiner I, Townsend CM: The role of surgery in the Zollinger–Ellison Syndrome. Ann Surg 197:594, 1983

15. Fox PS, Hofmann JW, DeCosse JJ, Wilson SD: The influence of total gastrectomy on survival in malignant ZE tumors. Ann Surg 180:558, 1974

16. Hancke S: Localization of hormone-producing gastrointestinal tumors by ultrasonic scanning. Scand J Gastroenterol 14(Supp 53):115, 1979

17. Deveney CW, Deveney KE, Stark D, Moss A, Stein S, Way LW: Resection of gastrinomas. Ann Surg 198:546, 1983

18. Damgaard-Pedersen K, Stage JG: Computed tomographic scanning in patients with ZES and carcinoid syndrome. Scand J Gastroenterol 14(Supp 53):117, 1979

19. Dunnick NR, Doppman JL, Mills S, McCarthy DM: Computed tomographic detection of non beta pancreatic islet cell tumors. Radiology 135:117, 1980

20. Roche A, Raisonnier A, Gillon-Savouvet M: Pancreatic venous sampling and arteriography in localizing insulinomas and gastrinomas: Procedure and results in 55 cases. Radiology 145:621, 1982

21. Mills SR, Doppman JL, Dunnick NR, McCarthy DM. Evaluation of angiography in ZES. Radiology 131:317, 1979

22. Burcharth F, Stage JB, Stadil F, Jensen L, Fischermann K. Localization of gastrinomas by transhepatic portal catheterization and gastrin assay. Gastroenterology 77:444, 1979

23. Stage JG, Stadil F. The clinical diagnosis of the ZES. Scand J Gastroenterol 14(Supp 53):79, 1979

24. McCarthy DM: The place of surgery in the ZES. N Eng J Med 302:1344, 1980

25. Malagelada JR, Edis AJ, Adson M, Van Heerden J, Go V: Medical and surgical options in the management of patients with gastrinoma. Gastroenterology 84:1524, 1983

26. Passaro E, Stabile BE. On gastrinomas and their management. Gastroenterology 84:1621, 1983

27. Stabile BE, Ippoliti AF, Walsh JH, Passaro E. Failure of histamine $H_2$-receptor antagonist therapy in ZES. Am J Surg 145:17, 1983
28. Bonfils S, Mignon M, Vallot T, Mayeur S: Use of ranitidine in the medical treatment of ZES. Scand J Gastroenterol 16:Supp 16:119, 1981
29. Richardson CT, Feldman M, McClelland RN, Dickerman RM, Kumpuris D, Fortran J: Effect of vagotomy in ZES. Gastroenterology 77:682, 1979
30. Barreras RF, Mack E, Goodfriend T, Damm M: Resection of gastrinoma in the ZES. Gastroenterology 82:953, 1982
31. Stabile B, Morrow DJ, Passaro E: The gastrinoma triangle: Operative implications. Am J Surg 147:25, 1984
32. Bonfils S, Landor JH, Mignon M, Hervoir P: Results of surgical management in 92 consecutive patients with ZES. Ann Surg 194:692, 1981
33. Brennan M, Jensen R, Wesley RA, Doppman JL, McCarthy DM: The role of surgery in patients with ZES (ZES) managed medically. Ann Surg 196:239, 1982
34. Friesen SR: Tumors of the endocrine pancreas. N Engl J Med 306:580, 1982
35. Moertel CG, Hanley JA, Johnson LA: Streptozocin alone compared with streptozocin plus fluorouracil in the treatment of advanced islet-cell carcinoma. N Engl J Med 303:1189, 1980
36. Friesen SR: Effect of total gastrectomy on the ZE tumor: Observation by second-look procedures. Surgery 62:609, 1967
37. Zollinger RM, Martin EW, Carey L, Sparks J, Minton JP: Observations on the postoperative tumor growth of certain islet cell tumors. Ann Surg 184:525, 1976
38. Graham RR: Quoted in Howland G, Campbell WR, Maltby EJ, Robinson WL: Dysinsulinism, convulsions and coma due to islet cell tumors of the pancreas with operation and cure. JAMA 93:674, 1929
39. Whipple AO: The surgical therapy of hyperinsulinism. J Int Chir 3:237, 1938
40. Yalow RS, Berson SA: Assay of plasma insulin in human subjects by immunologic methods. Nature 184:1648, 1959
41. Stefanini P, Carboni M, Patrassi N, Basoli A: Beta-Islet cell tumors of the pancreas: Results of a study on 1067 cases. Surgery 75:597, 1974
42. Carcassonne M, DeLarue A, Letourneau J: Surgical treatment of organic pancreatic hypoglycemia in the pediatric age. J Ped Surg 18:75, 1983
43. van Heerden JA, Edis AJ: Insulinoma: Diagnosis and management. Surg Rounds 3:42, 1980
44. Service FJ, Dale AJ, Elveback LR, Jiang N: Insulinoma: Clinical and diagnostic features of 60 consecutive cases. Mayo Clin Proc 51:417, 1976
45. Hsien-Chiu T, Wei-Jan W, Chu Y, Tung-Lua, L: Insulinoma: Experience in surgical treatment. Arch Surg 115:647, 1980
46. Galbut DL, Markowitz AM: Insulinoma: Diagnosis, surgical management and long term follow-up. Am J Surg 139:682, 1980
47. Roche A, Raisonnier A, Gillon-Savouret M: Pancreatic venous sampling and arteriography in localizing insulinomas and gastrinomas; Procedure and results in 55 cases. Radiology 145:621, 1982
48. Fulton RE, Sheedy PF, McIlrath D, Ferris DO: Pre-operative angiographic localization of insulin producing tumors of the pancreas. Am J Roentgenol 123:367, 1975
49. Ingemansson S, Kuhl C, Larsson LI, Lunderquist A, Lunoquist I: Localization of insulinomas and islet cell hyperplasias by pancreatic vein catheterization and insulin assay. Surg Gynec Obstetr 146:725, 1978
50. Modlin IM: Endocine tumors of the pancreas. Surg Gynecol Obstetr 149:751, 1979

51. LeQuesne LP, Nabarro JDN, Kurtz A, Zweig S: The management of insulin tumors of the pancreas. Br J Surg 66:373, 1979
52. Muir JJ, Offord K, van Heerden JA, Tinker JH, Endres SM: Glucose management in patients undergoing operation for insulinoma removal. Anesthesiology 59:371, 1983
53. Kaplan EL, Lee C: Recent advances in the diagnosis and treatment of insulinoma. Surg Clin North Am 59:119, 1979
54. Murray FT, Rae L, Langer B, Ambus U, Marliss EB, Nakhooda AF: Remission of hypoglycemia after partial resection of a metastatic islet cell tumor. Am J Surg 135:846, 1978
55. Stefanini P, Carboni M, Patrassi N, Basoli A: The surgical treatment of occult insulinomas: A review of the problem. Br. J. Surg. 61:1, 1974
56. Sigel B, Duarte B, Coelho J, Nyhus L, Baker R, Machi J: Localization of insulinomas of the pancreas at operation by real-time ultrasound scanning. Surg Gynecol Obstetr 156:145, 1983
57. Lane RJ, Coupland GA: Operative ultrasonic features of insulinoma. Am J Surg 144:585, 1982
58. Keaveny TV, Tawes R, Belzer FO: A new method for intraoperative indentification of insulinomas. Br J Surg 58:233, 1971
59. Turner RC, Lee EC, Morris PJ, Harris EA: Localization of insulinomas. Lancet 1:515, 1978
60. Edis AJ, McIlrath DC, van Heerden JA: Insulinoma: Current diagnosis and surgical management. Curr Prob Surg 13:1, 1976
61. Tuft GO, Edis AJ, Service FJ, Van Heerden JA: Plasma glucose monitoring during operation for insulinoma: A critical reappraisal. Surgery 88:351, 1980
62. Schwartz S, Horwitz DL, Zehfus B, Langer BE, Kaplan E: Continuous monitoring and control of plasma glucose during operation for removal of insulinomas. Surgery 85:702, 1979
63. Kudlow JE, Albisser AM, Angel A, Langer B, Yip CC, Zinman B, Stokes, E: Insulinoma resection facilitated by the artificial endocrine pancreas. Diabetes 27:774, 1978
64. Rich RH, Dehner CP, Okinaga K, Deeb LC, Ulstrom RA, Leonard AS: Surgical management of islet cell adenoma in infancy. Surgery 84:519, 1978
65. Becker SW, Kahn D, Rothman S: Cutaneous manifestations of internal malignant tumors. Arch Dermatol Syph 45:1069, 1942
66. McGavran MH, Unger RH, Recent L, Polk H, Kilo C, Levin M: A glucagon-secreting alpha-cell carcinoma of the pancreas. N Engl J Med 274:1408, 1966
67. Mallinson CN, Bloom SR, Warin AP, Salmon PR, Cox B: A glucagonoma syndrome. Lancet 2:1, 1974
68. Higgins GA: Pancreatic islet cell tumors: Insulinoma, gastrinoma, and glucagonoma. Surg Clin North Amer 59:131, 1979
69. Prinz RA, Badrinath K, Banerji M, Sparagana M, Dorsch T, Lawrence A: Operative and chemotherapeutic management of malignant glucagon-producing tumors. Surgery 90:713, 1981
70. Kessinger A, Lemon HM, Foley JF: The glucagonoma syndrome and its management. J Surg Oncol 9:419, 1977
71. Leichter SB: Clinical and metabolic aspects of glucagonoma. Medicine 59:100, 1980
72. Boden G, Owen O: Familial hyperglucagonemia: An autosomal dominant disorder. N Engl J Med 296:534, 1977
73. Ingemansson S., Holst JJ et al: Localization of glucagonomas by catheterization of the pancreatic veins and with glucagon assay. Surg Gynecol Obstet 145:509, 1977

74. Higgins GA, Recant L, Fischman AB: The glucagonoma syndrome: Surgically curable diabetes. Am J Surg 137:142, 1979

75. Lokich J, Anderson N et al: Pancreatic alpha cell tumors: Case report and review of the literature. Cancer 45:2675, 1980

76. Montenegro F, Lawrence GD, Macon W, Ross C: Metastatic glucagonoma: Improvement after surgical debulking. Am J Surg 139:424, 1980

77. Bordi C, Ravazzola M, Baetens D, Gordon P, Unger R, Orci L: A study of glucagonoma by light and electron microscopy and immunofluorescence. Diabetes 28:925, 1979

78. Friesen SR, Hermreck AS, Mantz FA: Glucagon, gastrin, and carcinoid tumors of the duodenum, pancreas, and stomach: Polypeptide "APUDomas" of the foregut. Am J Surg 129:90, 1974

79. Strauss GM, Weitzman SA, Aoki TT: Dimethyltriazenoimidazole carboxamide therapy of malignant glucagonoma. Ann Int Med 90:57, 1979

80. Brazeau P, Burgus R, Vale W, Ling N, Guillemain R: Hypothalamic polypeptide that inhibits the secretion of immunoreactive pituitary growth hormone. Science 179:77, 1973

81. Polak JM, Pearse AGE, Grimeius L, Bloom SR, Arimura A: GH release inhibiting hormone (GH-RIH) in GI and pancreatic D cells. Lancet 1:1220, 1975

82. Ganda OP, Weir GC, Soeldner JS, et al: "Somatostatinoma": A somatostatin containing tumor of the endocrine pancreas. N Engl J Med 296:963–967, 1977

83. Larsson LI, Hirsch MA, Holst JJ, Kuhl C, Lundquist G, and Rehfeld JF: Pancreatic somatostatinoma: Clinical features and implications. Lancet 1:666, 1977

84. Kelly TR: Pancreatic somatostatinoma. Am J Surg 146:671, 1983

85. Sakazaki S, Umeyama K, Nakagawa H, Hashimoto H, Kamino K, Mitsuhashi T, Yamaguchi K: Pancreatic somatostatinoma. Am J Surg 146:674, 1983

86. Krejs GJ, Orci L, Conlon JM, Ravazzola M, Davis, GR, Unger RH: Somatostatinoma syndrome: Biochemical, morphologic and clinical features. N Engl J Med 301:285, 1979

87. Bloom SR, Polak JM: Glucagonomas, VIPomas, and somatostatinomas. J Clin Endocrinol Metab 9:285, 1980

88. Kaneko H, Yanaihara N, Ito S, Kusumoto Y, Fujita T, Ishihawas, Sumida T, Sekiya M: Somatostatinoma of the duodenum. Cancer 44:2273, 1979

89. Stacpoole PW, Kasselberg AG, Berelowitz M, Chey W: Somatostatinoma syndrome: Does a clinical entity exist? Acta Endocrinol 102:80, 1983

90. Verner JV, Morrison AB: Islet cell tumor and a syndrome of refractory watery diarrhea and hypokalemia. Am J Med 25:374, 1958

91. Verner JV, Morrison AB: Endocrine pancreatic islet disease with diarrhea. Arch Int Med 133:492, 1974

92. Long RG, Bryant MG, Mitchell SJ, Adrian TE, Polak JM, Bloom SR: Clinicopathological study of pancreatic and ganglioneuroblastoma tumors secreting vasoactive intestinal polypeptide (VIPomas). Br Med J 282:1767, 1981

93. Jaffe BM, Condon S: Prostaglandins E and F in endocrine diarrheogenic syndromes. Ann Surg 184:516, 1976

94. Tomita T, Kimmel JR, Friesen SR, Mantz FA: Pancreatic polypeptide cell hyperplasia with and without watery diarrhea syndrome. J Surg Oncol 14:11, 1980

95. Schwartz TW: Pancreatic polypeptide (PP) and endocrine tumours of the pancreas. Scand J Gastroenterol 14, Suppl 53:93–100, 1979

96. Modlin IM, Bloom SR, Mitchell SJ: Experimental evidence for vasoactive intestinal

polypeptide as the cause of the watery diarrhea syndrome. Gastroenterology 75:1051, 1978

97. Ebeid AM, Murray PD, Fischer JE: Vasoactive intestinal polypeptide and the watery diarrhea syndrome. Ann Surg 187:411, 1978

98. Bloom SR: Vasoactive intestinal polypeptide and watery diarrhea. p. 583. In Gut Hormones. Bloom SR, Ed. New York: Churchill Livingstone, 1978

99. Yamada T: Secretory tumors of the pancreas. p. 1528. In Gastrointestinal Disease. Sleisenger M, Fordtran J, Eds. Philadelphia: WB Saunders, 1983

100. Hoover HC: Endocrine tumors of the pancreas. p. 126. In Surgery of the Alimentary Tract, Shachelford RT, Zuidema GD, Eds. Philadelphia: WB Saunders, 1983

101. Jaffe BM, Kopen DF, DeSchryver-Keskemeti K, Gingerich RL, Greider M: Indomethacin-Responsive Pancreatic Cholera. N Engl J Med 297:817, 1977

102. Capella C, Polak JM, Buffa R, Tapia F, Heitz P, Usselini L, Bloom SR, Solcia E: Morphologic patterns and diagnostic criteria for VIP-producing endocrine tumors. Cancer 52:1860, 1983

103. Nagorney DM, Bloom SR, Polak J, Blumgart LH: Resolution of recurrent Verner–Morrison Syndrome by resection of metastatic VIPoma. Surgery 93:348, 1983

104. Kahn CR, Levy AG, Gardner JD, Miller JV, Gorden P, Schein P: Pancreatic cholera: Beneficial effects of therapy with streptozotocin. N Engl J Med 292:941, 1975

105. Oberndorfer S: Karzinoide: Tumoren des Dunndaums. Frankfurt Z Pathol 1:426, 1907

106. Thorson A: Studies on carcinoid disease. Acta Med Scand Supp 134:1, 1963

107. Williams ED, Sandler M: The classification of carcinoid tumors. Lancet 1:238, 1963

108. Wareing TH, Sawyers JL: Carcinoids and the carcinoid syndrome. Am J Surg 145:769, 1983

109. Aranha G, Greenlee H: Surgical management of carcinoid tumors of the gastrointestinal tract. Am Surg 46:429, 1980

110. Kawlessar OD: The carcinoid syndrome. p. 1250. In Gastrointestinal Disease, Sleisenger M, Fordtran J, Eds.: Philadelphia: WB Saunders, 1983

111. Beaton H, Homan W, Dineen P: Gastrointestinal carcinoids and the malignant carcinoid syndrome. Surg Gynecol Obstet 152:268, 1981

112. Strodel WE, Talpos G, Eckhauser F, Thompson N: Surgical therapy for small-bowel carcinoid tumors. Arch Surg 118:391, 1983

113. Feldman JM, Jones RS: Carcinoid syndrome from gastrointestinal carcinoids without liver metastasis. Ann Surg 196:33, 1982

114. Kellum JM, Jaffe BM: Validation and application of a radioimmunoassay for serotonin. Gastroenterology 70:516, 1976

115. Tilson MD: Carcinoid syndrome. Surg Clin North Am 54:409, 1974

116. Warner TF, O'Reilly G, Power LH: Carcinoid diathesis of the ileum. Cancer 43:1900, 1979

117. Peck JJ, Shields AB, Boyden AM, Dworkin LA, Nadal JW: Carcinoid tumors of the ileum. Am J Surg 146:124, 1983

118. Condon R: Unusual disorders of the stomach. p. 557. In: Surgery of the Stomach, Nyhus CM, Wastell, C, Eds. 3rd Edition, Boston: Little Brown, 1977

119. Goodwin JD: Carcinoid tumors: An analysis of 2837 cases. Cancer 36:560, 1975

120. Lasson A, Alwmark A, Nobin A, Sundler F: Endocrine tumors of the duodenum. Ann Surg 197:393, 1983

121. Morgan JG, Marks C, Hearn D: Carcinoid tumors of the gastrointestinal tract. Ann Surg 180:720, 1974

122. Moertel CG, Sauer G, Dockerty MB, Baggenstoss AH: Life history of carcinoid tumors of the small intestine. Cancer 14:901, 1961

123. Eckhauser FE, Argenta LC, Strodel WE, Wheeler RH, Bull F, Appelman HD, Thompson N: Mesenteric angiopathy, intestinal gangrene, and midgut carcinoids. Surgery 90:720, 1981

124. Davis Z, Moertel CG, McIlrath DC: The malignant carcinoid syndrome. Surg. Gynecol Obstet 137:637, 1973

125. Welch JP, Malt RA: Management of carcinoid tumors of the gastrointestinal tract. Surg Gynecol Obstet 145:223, 1977

126. Kirkegaard P, Hjortrup A, Halse C, Luke M, Christiansen J: Long-term results of surgery for carcinoid tumors of the gastrointestinal tract. Acta Chir Scand 147:693, 1981

127. Gillett DJ, Smith RC: Treatment of the carcinoid syndrome by hemihepatectomy and radical excision of the primary lesion. Am J Surg 128:95, 1974

128. Martin JK, Moertel CG, Adson M, Schutt AJ: Surgical treatment of functioning metastatic carcinoid tumors. Arch Surg 118:537, 1983

129. Idema AA, Niermeyer P, Oldhoff J: Hepatic dearterialization for carcinoid syndrome due to liver metastases. Arch Chir Neerl 29:125, 1977

130. Helmer RE, Morettin LB, Costanzi JJ: Hepatic artery occlusion with perfusion in the treatment of the carcinoid syndrome. Oncology 38:361, 1981

131. Moertel CG, Dockerty MB, Judd ES: Carcinoid tumors of the vermiform appendix. Cancer 21:270, 1968

132. Dent TL, Batsakis JG, Lindenauer SM: Carcinoid tumors of the appendix. Surgery 73:828, 1973

133. Syracuse DC, Perzin KH, Price JB, Wiebel PD, Mesa-Tejada, R: Carcinoid tumors of the appendix: Mesoappendiceal extension and nodal metastases. Ann Surg 190:58, 1979

134. Berardi RS: Carcinoid tumors of the colon (exclusive of the rectum): Review of the literature. Dis Colon Rectum 15:383, 1972

135. Wilson H, Cheek RC: Carcinoid tumors. In: Current Problems in Surgery, Chicago: Yearbook Medical Publishers, 1970

136. Peskin GW, Orloff MJ. A clinical study of 25 patients with carcinoid tumors of the rectum. Surg Gynecol Obstet 109:673, 1959

137. Orloff MJ: Carcinoid tumors of the rectum. Cancer 28:175, 1971

# Index

Note: Page numbers followed by *f* denote figures; those followed by *t* denote tables